Pharmacokinetics

for the

Non-mathematical

Pharmacokinetics for the Non-mathematical

by

D. W. A. Bourne
Department of Pharmacy, University of Queensland, Australia

E. J. Triggs
Department of Pharmacy, University of Queensland, Australia

and

M. J. Eadie
Department of Medicine, University of Queensland, Australia

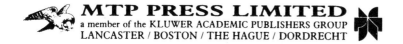
MTP PRESS LIMITED
a member of the KLUWER ACADEMIC PUBLISHERS GROUP
LANCASTER / BOSTON / THE HAGUE / DORDRECHT

Published in the UK and Europe by
MTP Press Limited
Falcon House
Lancaster, England

British Library Cataloguing in Publication Data
Bourne, David W. A.
    Pharmacokinetics for the non-mathematical.
    1. Pharmacokinetics
    I. Title   II. Triggs, Edward J.   III. Eadie, Mervyn J.
    615'.7   RM301.5
    ISBN 0-85200-712-4

Published in the USA by
MTP Press
A division of Kluwer Boston Inc.
190 Old Derby Street
Hingham, MA 02043, USA

Library of Congress Cataloging-in-Publication Data
Bourne, D. (David), 1946-
    Pharmacokinetics for the non-mathematical.
    Includes bibliographies and index.
    1. Pharmacokinetics.   I. Triggs, E. J. (Edward J.),
1942-   .   II. Eadie, Mervyn, J.   III. Title.
[DNLM: 1. Drugs–metabolism.   2. Kinetics.   QV 38 B775p]
RM301.5.B68   1986   615'.7   85-29752
ISBN 0-85200-712-4

Photosetting by Titus Wilson, Kendal, Cumbria
Printed in Great Britain by Butler & Tanner Limited
Frome and London

Contents

Preface

Several contemporary books on pharmacokinetics are available. Each has its particular merits, and each is most helpful in its own way. How can another book on the topic be justified?

Pharmacokinetic knowledge has had a very considerable influence on the thinking of recent pharmacy graduates. Unfortunately, it does not seem to have had an equal impact on the thinking of medical graduates. If the concepts of pharmacokinetics are valid, they should be a great help to those who are legally entitled to prescribe drugs. However, up to the present these concepts, if they have been accepted at all in medical practice, have often been received almost reluctantly and have sometimes been employed rather uncritically. Assuming that the concepts of pharmacokinetics are indeed valid, the relative failure, so far, of a potentially very useful tool to have a greater impact on contemporary medical thought and practice may have several explanations. For instance, the insights provided by applying pharmacokinetic principles in the clinical situation may have proved disturbing to the way of thinking of an older generation of clinicians. Additionally, the insights may have been seen merely as providing a rationale for existing and clinically satisfactory patterns of drug use (though accumulating experience suggests that pharmacokinetic insights often lead to altered and improved ways of using drugs). However, we suspect that the relative reluctance of the medical profession to make greater use of pharmacokinetic thinking has often stemmed from the way pharmacokinetic knowledge itself has been presented.

Some presentations of pharmacokinetics have been highly simplistic in terms of anatomy and physiology. Such presentations tend to be seen as rather unreal by clinicians, who have a well developed awareness of the structure and function of the human body and of biological variability. Other presentations are highly mathematical in their content. Medical graduates generally are not comfortable with mathematical, and particularly with algebraic, thinking. They tend to suspect that such highly mathematical approaches imply an unrealistic level of precision for any analysis of biological data. Further, the clinical examples often cited to convince the reader of the usefulness of their approach, frequently appear to the practising clinician as somewhat contrived, and implausible in the real life situation. They convey to the clinician's sense of physiological variation and human perversity, an impression of unreasonably precise and perhaps potentially dangerous prediction. In general, pharmacokinetic texts have not provided a very realistic translation of certain kinetic concepts into anatomical and physiological terms. It may well be that such a translation is not yet possible. However, the very acknowledgement of this fact might make the clinician more sympathetic to the worth of pharmacokinetics, and might enhance the intellectual stature of the discipline in his eyes. Even for those clinicians who sense the potential practical utility of pharmacokinetics, and wish to carry out pharmacokinetic analysis on their own data, there is the problem of finding adequate information in a single book about 'how to do it' in a form which they can use immediately. It is almost as though there has been a conspiracy to tantalize the clinician with the prospect of the wondrous data he might be able to obtain if he had access to a large computer and if someone else already had the appropriate program running on it, but to conceal from him how he could do his own pharmacokinetics fairly simply and cheaply, working at a level of exactness consistent with the accuracy of the data he is likely to obtain from his patients.

In the present book we have attempted to overcome to some extent what we have seen as shortcomings in the way the subject of pharmacokinetics has often been presented. We have tried to restrict algebra and mathematics to a minimum and have not always attempted to develop a logical consecutive mathematical system of reasoning. Rather, we have preferred at times to ask the reader to take certain mathematical statements on trust (but telling him when this is done). Where possible, mathematical ideas have been expressed in the form of graphs, since most medical graduates seem more comfortable interpreting graphs than equations. Throughout the book we have attempted a critical correlation of pharmacokinetic concepts with the level of anatomical and physiological knowledge one might expect of a medical graduate, and we have tried not to let the interpretation of pharmacokinetic ideas and the predictions drawn from them outrun the clinician's experience of what is likely to occur in a diseased state. We have been at some pains to distinguish that which is predicted from that which is established by observation. At the same time we have attempted to show how the predictions may be put to the test and, if proved correct, may later come to alter and enhance clinical practice. We have tried to show the clinician how he might carry out his own pharmacokinetic analyses of data with simple techniques using graph paper and hand-held calculators. In addition, bearing in mind the increasing availability of comparatively cheap 'home' microcomputers, we have also attempted to provide the clinician with access to 'software' that will allow him to carry out his own pharmacokinetic calculation at a quite reasonable level of sophistication and with a precision in keeping with the precision of the data he is likely to be able to collect from his patients (if he has access to a laboratory which can measure drugs at the concentrations at which they occur in clinical practice).

Thus we have tried to write a short, reasonably critical book on pharmacokinetics directed towards the interests and needs of medical students and medical graduates. Possibly the book may also provide some insights of value for students of pharmacy, dentistry, veterinary science and pharmacology. We hope it will lead some who practise medicine, or will soon practise it, to a heightened awareness of how pharmacokinetic thinking may make drug therapy more rational, more effective and safer.

D. W. A. Bourne
E. J. Triggs
and
M. J. Eadie

1
The rationale and use of pharmacokinetics

In nearly all instances drugs appear to produce their effects in man and other animals by forming bonds with various endogenous biological molecules. This bonding then sets in train further chemical events which find expression as the pharmacological action (or actions) of the drug. The processes of drug–receptor bonding, and the subsequent molecular events which transduce this interaction into the discernable 'actions' of the drug, are embraced by the term *pharmacodynamics*. In contrast, the term *pharmacokinetics* refers to those processes by which the drug enters the body, is moved around within the body (and thus reaches its sites of action), and is eliminated from the body (thus terminating any action it has in its own right). Thus pharmacokinetics embraces the (1) absorption, (2) distribution, and (3) elimination (by metabolic biotransformation and/or excretion of the unchanged compound) of drugs, but not their action. Distribution and elimination are sometimes referred to collectively in the single term 'disposition'. The word *pharmacokinetics* is often used in a more restricted sense than that above. It then refers only to the mathematical analysis of the processes of drug absorption, distribution and elimination. It is in this latter sense that the word *pharmacokinetics* will be used from here on in this book.

If such mathematical procedures are to prove clinically relevant, at the very least they should be able to assist the clinician in his use of drugs. The clinician's chief purpose in using drugs is to achieve the therapeutic benefit desired without producing an unacceptable level of unwanted effects. The clinician's concern thus lies primarily in the pharmacodynamics of the drugs he uses. The question then arises: how can pharmacokinetics assist the clinician in his concern with pharmacodynamic matters?

Depending on the drug and the circumstances under consideration, there may be one or more answers to this question. The most widely applicable answer is the claim that pharmacokinetic knowledge helps the clinician predict the likely time course and extent of the effect of a given dose of a drug in a given individual. This answer is valid even in those occasional instances when the action of the drug in question can be measured immediately and conveniently, e.g. the regulation of heart rate in cardiac arrhythmia, the control of blood glucose concentration in diabetes mellitus, the decrease of prothrombin activity in thromboembolic vascular disease and the reduction of airways resistance in asthma. Even in these circumstances it is still useful to the clinician to know approximately when the maximum effect of a drug dose may be expected. He may then ascertain whether, at that time, benefit still outweighs undesired effects without the necessity of carrying out sequential measurements of the relevant drug actions. It is also helpful for the clinician to know in advance when the effect of a given dose of a drug is likely to cease, so that a second dose may be given at an appropriate time.

A second answer arises in relation to drugs whose actions are not readily quantified and/or have clinical effects which may not be obvious until some time after the drug initiates its biochemical effects. Thus in antimicrobial chemotherapy a dose of an antibiotic may kill or inactivate the responsible organisms within a few hours. However, the clinician may not be sure that he has prescribed adequate therapy for another 2 or 3 days, until resolution of various aspects of the inflammatory process produced by the infection has had time to become clinically apparent. In such a situation knowledge of the minimum inhibitory concentration for the chemotherapeutic agent towards the causative micro-organism, and use of pharmacokinetic information concerning the agent's disposition will enable calculation of the likely range of concentrations of the agent that will be achieved in the relevant body fluid. This knowledge can give the clinician reasonable grounds for expecting that he has prescribed adequate therapy, even at the outset of treatment. Drugs are sometimes given to prevent disorders which occur episodically, at irregular and often unpredictable intervals (as in epilepsy or migraine). In such cases if the relation between drug effects and drug concentrations in accessible body fluids is known, pharmacokinetic calculations can be used to determine whether a potentially suitable drug dosage is being used, without having to await the clinical response revealed by the passage of time.

How is it possible for pharmacokinetic information to be used in these ways to, as it were, anticipate the course of a drug's pharmacodynamics? The answer lies in considering events at the interface between pharmacokinetics and pharmacodynamics, i.e. the binding of drug molecules to receptors, and in considering the way in which drug molecules become distributed through the body.

DRUG–RECEPTOR INTERACTIONS

Receptor events

The term 'receptor' has sometimes been applied to all tissue molecules which form chemical bonds with drug molecules. Here the term 'receptor' is used more restrictively. It refers only to those binding sites at which the bonding leads to further chemical events which become manifest as pharmacological actions of the drug, both desired and undesired. The word 'acceptor' may be used to refer to those binding sites at which the bonding leads to no pharmacological effect.

Reversible bonding

Bonding between drug and receptor is, in most instances, non-covalent (i.e. it is electrostatic, involving ionic, dipole–dipole or hydrogen bonding). Such bonding tends to be readily reversible under physiological conditions. In such instances, the degree of drug action generally appears proportionate to the number of receptor molecules bonded to drug molecules at any given time. This is the basis of the receptor 'occupancy' hypothesis, though in relation to this hypothesis quantitative effects of the bonding may be influenced by some receptors being in an inactive state when drug molecules bond to them. In contrast to this situation, drug action occasionally appears proportionate to the rate at which drug molecules bond to receptors. This rate is determined by the rate at which previously formed drug–receptor combinations break down, leaving receptors available for further bonding to other drug molecules. In either situation the concentration of drug molecules in the region of receptors (in the so-called 'biophase') is a determinant of the rate and number of drug–receptor bondings. Drug concentration in the biophase thus tends to determine quantitative aspects of drug action. If one could measure drug concentrations in the biophase one would have a measure of drug effect, even if that effect could not readily be measured directly and even if the effect was not immediately detectable, because of delay in the translation of drug–receptor bonding into discernible actions.

There is considerable contemporary interest in the study of drug–receptor interactions. It seems likely that this study will throw considerable additional light on quantitative considerations at the drug–receptor interface. The above simplistic account of drug–receptor events may need substantial modification in the future. Further, it may be wise to sound a note of caution about the interpretation of some of the earlier drug binding studies. Contemporary biochemical methodology makes it comparatively easy to demonstrate bonding between drug molecules and tissue molecules. This demonstration is not proof that the binding sites are necessarily receptor sites, if the word 'receptor' is used restrictively to refer to tissue molecules where bonding is ultimately transduced into pharmacological activity. Sometimes one can be reasonably sure that the binding of a drug to its actual receptors has been studied, because the number of bindings was directly proportional to a biochemical change consequent on the binding, and this biochemical change is known to mediate the action of the drug, e.g. formation of cyclic adenosine monophosphate following the attachment of noradrenaline to certain types of β-adrenoceptors. Sometimes the evidence that a drug has bound to its receptors is less direct, and therefore less compelling. Thus the binding of a series of congeneric drug molecules may be shown to parallel the known potencies of these drugs towards the actions mediated by the receptor studied. Unfortunately at times in the past, it appears to have been assumed that any tissue molecule to which a drug binds is necessarily a receptor for that drug. Until quantitative aspects of drug–receptor bonding have been subjected to further critical experimental study it may be unwise to attempt to refine interpretation of events at the pharmacokinetic–pharmacodynamic interface. One as yet has little secure basis for going beyond the generalization that drug effect is likely to prove proportionate to drug concentration in the biophase. Even here there should be the proviso that, as drug concentration in the biophase rises, there must come a stage at which maximum receptor occupancy (and maximum drug effect) occurs, since there must be a finite number of receptors in the body. There is now reasonably good evidence that receptor numbers in a given organism may not be static, but may alter as a consequence of physiological factors or as a result of drug–receptor bonding itself. This alteration may change the biophase drug concentration–pharmacological response relationship, particularly at higher drug concentrations, and thus vary the upper limits of the pharmacological response.

The expected relationship between biophase drug concentration and biological effect for a reversibly-bonded drug might be expected to resem-

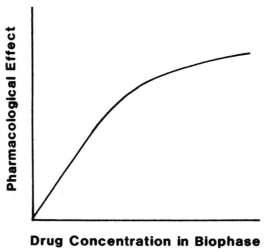

Drug Concentration in Biophase

Figure 1.1 Relation between pharmacological effect and drug concentration in biophase for a reversibly bound drug

ble that shown in Figure 1.1. A similar appearance should also apply if there were a rate-limiting biochemical step at some stage between drug–receptor binding and the appearance of the pharmacological action of the drug, though here, of course, it would not be the drug–receptor bonding that set the limit to the pharmacological effect.

Irreversible bonding

In the previous section we have been considering drug–receptor bonding when the bonding is readily reversible under physiological conditions. But what happens when the bonding is covalent, and essentially irreversible

4

under physiological circumstances unless there is an enzyme present which can catalyse bond cleavage? When drug concentration rises in the biophase, previously unoccupied receptors will become occupied by drug molecules, and drug action will increase in extent. When drug concentration in the biophase subsequently falls, unlike the situation in reversible bonding, receptors already occupied will not become vacant. Therefore drug action will not diminish. Drug action will continue, even when no drug remains in the biophase, until the occupied receptors are themselves degraded and replaced, or until some subsequent stage in the biochemical events that transduce the drug–receptor bonding into the drug's action is interrupted. The pharmacokinetics of an irreversibly-bound drug such as the monoamine oxidase inhibitor phenelzine (i.e. its absorption, distribution and elimination) can be interpreted mathematically, and its concentrations elsewhere can be related to drug concentration in the biophase. However, the biophase concentrations of irreversibly-bound drugs show no simple consistent

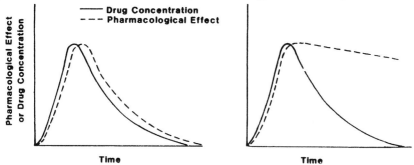

Figure 1.2 Time courses of drug concentrations (continuous line) and pharmacological effects (broken lines) for reversibly bound (left half) and irreversibly bound (right half) drugs

direct relationship to biological effect (Figure 1.2). This is unlike the situation for the drug with reversible bonding to receptors (for which drug concentration in the biophase tends to be proportionate to the pharmacological effect of the drug, at least over a certain concentration range). Given the present state of knowledge it would be very difficult to determine any sort of simple exact mathematical equivalence between biophase concentrations of irreversibly-bound drugs and pharmacological effects. Drug effects are the clinician's prime concern. Therefore, pharmacokinetics has less to offer the clinician in the case of irreversibly-bound drugs than in the much more common situation of reversible drug–receptor bonding. Admittedly, if one knew the time course of the degradation of drug–receptor complexes, and the rate of new receptor synthesis, it should be possible to define a mathematical relationship between biophase drug concentration and biological effect for irreversibly-bound drugs. However, the requisite knowledge is not yet available, and even if it were the mathematics involved might prove rather formidable, and perhaps too complex to be used in practice.

Drug concentrations in the biophase

Pharmacokinetics is made a practical possibility by the ability to measure drugs at the concentrations at which they are found in the human body during the course of therapy. Without the ability to carry out such concentration measurements pharmacokinetics could be only a theoretical exercise. It might be illuminating conceptually, but it would be difficult to apply in the concrete situation of the individual patient prescribed a drug.

The argument has been developed above for measuring drug concentration in the biophase as an often valid indication of the likely degree of pharmacological effect produced by a drug. That may well be so, but is it practicable to measure drug concentration in the biophase? Analytical methodology has achieved sufficient sophistication for it to be nearly always possible to measure drugs with adequate specificity and sensitivity at the concentrations at which they occur in the biophase. Therefore the answer to the question posed above would usually be yes, so long as the anatomical location of the biophase was known, and samples could be collected from this locale. Presumably the biophase would comprise that portion of body water in close proximity to the drugs receptors and with free access to them. But what are the dimensions of close proximity? And are the relevant drug receptors restricted to one anatomical site in the body, or must multiple, different biophases at different receptor sites, possibly in different organs and tissues, be sampled? And can we ever know where the relevant receptors are for all drugs, so that we can know where to sample the biophase? Even if we could answer these questions (and sometimes we cannot) we may still be left in a situation that is ethically and practically impossible, i.e. of having to biopsy quite inaccessible sites in several parts of the body to obtain the data sought, with some of these biopsies carrying a much greater hazard than the disease being treated. Thus, if a phenothiazine drug (a dopamine antagonist) were used to treat nausea, the relevant biophase would be that of the chemoreceptor trigger zone of the medulla oblongata. Obtaining a sample from this region would require major neurosurgery and would carry quite prohibitive dangers. And since one might also be concerned about the extrapyramidal unwanted effects of the therapy, the biophase in the corpus striatum should also be studied. Again such sampling would involve quite unacceptable hazards.

Except in rare instances, it is not practicable to measure drug concentration in the biophase(s), simply because it would be completely unreasonable to attempt to sample this portion of body water. Does the possibility of applying pharmacokinetics thus founder on this simple issue of practicality and ethics? There is, in fact, a solution to the dilemma, a solution based on knowledge of how a drug becomes distributed throughout the body. This solution resolves the ethical problem and offers an advantage of simplicity. However, it sacrifices something of the precision that might accrue from measurements made on the drug in its actual biophase, or biophases.

DRUG DISTRIBUTION IN THE BODY

Spatial pattern

Drug molecules are rarely moved through cell membranes by active or

6

facilitated transport. Much more often their movement within the body occurs by virtue of passive transfer along concentration gradients. Therefore in nearly all instances the spatial pattern of drug distribution within the body tends to be determined by (1) drug solubility in various body fluids and in the component molecules of tissues, particularly the molecules in cell membranes, (2) bonding of drug molecules to various molecules (not only to receptor molecules) in body fluids and in cell membranes, and (3) movement of body fluids, particularly the blood and interstitial fluids.

Drug distribution within the body at a particular moment can be schematized as a series of concentration equilibria (Figure 1.3).

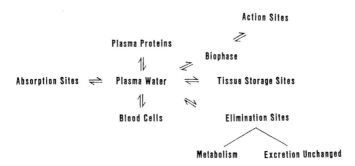

Figure 1.3 Scheme of the equilibria involved in drug distribution within the body

In the interests of simplicity the scheme in Figure 1.3 may not have made certain possibilities as clear as it might. Thus for the one drug there may be multiple different receptor sites, and a different biophase for each type of receptor site, and some (or all) of the biophases may be part of interstitial water (or even of plasma water). The scheme indicates that, at any moment, drug concentration in the biophase (or biophases) is related, through one or more concentration equilibria, to drug concentration in plasma (and the latter is nearly always readily measurable). This comes about as follows. In most instances, drug in the biophase(s) will be separated from drug in plasma water by one or more lipid membranes; transfer of drug molecules through these membranes is almost always a passive process, the rate of which is proportionate to the drug concentration gradient. Therefore, drug concentration in plasma water should vary in proportion to drug concentrations in the various biophases. Even if there are multiple biophases in the body, though the concentration equilibrium between each biophase and plasma water may differ from the next, the concentration of the drug in plasma water throughout the body (a comparatively uniform concentration because of intravascular mixing and the rapidity of the circulation) will still provide a single common measure of (the different) drug concentrations in the biophases. Therefore, drug concentration in plasma water provides an index of all the effects of a given drug (so long as the drug is one that binds reversibly to receptors, as most drugs do, and all available receptor sites are not saturated with drug). Thus measurement of drug concentration in plasma water yields information about the likely quantitative effects of reversibly bound drugs.

In practice it is often rather cumbersome to measure drug concentrations in plasma water, because of the laboratory processes (dialysis, ultrafiltration) involved in separating plasma water from plasma proteins. Therefore, in view of the further reversible concentration equilibria between drug molecules in plasma water, and those bound to plasma proteins (Figure 1.3), drug concentrations are usually measured in whole plasma. Whole plasma drug concentrations are taken as a measure of biophase drug concentrations. However, it should be realized that plasma proteins also have a finite number of sites to which drug molecules can bind. Consequently, the relationship between concentrations of drug bound to plasma proteins and drug free in plasma water may not necessarily be linear over a wide range of drug concentrations. This non-linearity may lead to error in attempting to correlate whole plasma drug concentration data with clinical effects of the drug in question. When drug concentration in whole plasma is used as a measure of the likely pharmacological effect of a drug it should be realized that the various concentration equilibria between various zones of the body condensed into this equivalence involve at least two stages at which the concentration relationships are not necessarily simple, direct proportional ones. These two stages are at the plasma protein–plasma water interface, and at the drug–receptor interface. With this qualification, whole plasma drug levels at a given moment do provide a measure of the pharmacological effect of a drug that is reversibly bound to its receptors and which is not subject to active or facilitated transport through biological membranes.

Quantitative aspects of drug distribution may change with time after dose intake, largely as a result of the ongoing processes of drug absorption and drug elimination. Thus far, drug distribution has been dealt with as though it were a static, unchanging event. The time factor in drug distribution should now be considered, for pharmacokinetics involves not merely the interpretation of drug concentrations within the body at a particular moment, but also the interpretation of their time courses.

Temporal pattern

After a drug dose is given by any route other than the intravenous one, the drug concentration in plasma rises until the time when the amount of drug being absorbed in unit time falls below the amount being eliminated over the same period. After this time plasma drug concentration falls progressively until the next drug dose is taken. Drug concentrations in the biophase will tend to follow the time course of drug concentrations in plasma, but there may be an appreciable time lag between the two. This lag time is determined by the rate and extent of the circulation to various regions of the body, the rates of transfer of drug molecules across the various biological membranes intervening between the circulation and the biophase and by binding equilibria rates. This delay may distort the quantitative constancy of the static relationship between plasma and bio-

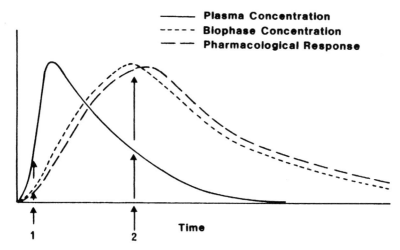

Figure 1.4 Time course of drug concentrations in plasma and the biophase after a drug dose. At times 1 and 2 the same plasma drug concentrations are associated with very different drug concentrations in the biophase and with different biological effects. However, in the postdistribution phase (well after 2), when the drug has achieved its definitive distribution throughout the body, the ratio between plasma and biophase drug concentrations becomes relatively constant until the next dose is taken

phase drug concentrations discussed in the preceding section. As indicated in the legend to Figure 1.4, after enough time has elapsed following a drug dose for drug distribution to have attained its definitive pattern, the ratio between plasma and biophase drug concentrations should remain reasonably constant until the next dose is given. During the earlier distributional phase there may be a higher ratio of plasma to biophase drug concentrations, relative to the postdistributive value of this ratio. This higher value is a consequence of the more restricted but increasing extent of distribution of the drug in the body as the distribution phase proceeds.

Thus the arguments developed relating plasma drug concentration to pharmacological effect should be subjected to the caveat that they apply more closely after a drug has achieved its final distribution pattern in the body.

THE POSSIBILITY OF MATHEMATICAL PHARMACOKINETICS AND ITS VALUE

So far we have developed a semiquantitative argument. This argument attempts to show that, with the presence of a drug in the body, for the majority of drugs (those that appear to bind reversibly to their receptors and are transported passively across plasma membranes) there is a relationship, though not necessarily a constant proportionality, between plasma drug level and potential pharmacological effect of the drug. Is it feasible to define such a relationship with greater mathematical precision? Would such a mathematical description have any practical value?

It will be shown in subsequent chapters that, by virtue of making a number of physiologically reasonable assumptions and simplifications, it is possible to develop mathematical descriptions of the time courses of the presence of drugs in the body. This type of mathematical analysis is applicable to the type of plasma level vs. time data that it is feasible to collect from man. The more adequately the plasma level data are described in terms of physiological and anatomical reality, the more complicated the mathematics required tend to be, but the more reliable are the predictions that can be drawn from the findings, always assuming that the mathematics themselves can be worked out. Because the mathematical descriptions are developed in relation to the particular range of drug concentrations studied, it is always possible that the description, though valid within this concentration range, may prove inadequate if applied to a wider concentration range.

And to what use can the mathematical descriptions be put? In what ways can they help the clinician?

(1) The analysis of pharmacokinetic data and the predictions drawn from this analysis can provide additional insights into what appears to happen to drugs within the body.

(2) So long as the range of plasma drug concentrations associated with a particular pharmacological effect is known, pharmacokinetic data drawn from the population (and preferably, if possible, from the individual in question) can be applied to the individual to give the prescriber a better basis for determining:

(a) the appropriate drug dose to gain a desired effect,

(b) the appropriate dosage interval, if the drug is to be given in repeated dosage,

(c) the likely time course of the drug's biological effect after each dose, including the time when the maximum effect can be expected, and the time when the effect should have worn off.

By use of this information therapeutic regimes may be rationalized, often simplified and yet made more effective.

(3) Pharmacokinetic awareness may assist in the recognition and interpretation of the mechanism of drug–drug interactions when more than one drug is taken by a patient, and may help in the recognition of possible adverse effects of drugs.

(4) The numerical values of pharmacokinetic data allow a great deal of information about drugs to be contained and stored in a very concise form. The values of standard pharmacokinetic parameters become, in effect, a code which, if understood, gives the clinician access to drug information stored in a readily portable form. He can then use this information for the purposes set down immediately above (1, 2 and 3).

THE VALIDITY OF PHARMACOKINETICS

Pharmacokinetics has had a considerable effect in enhancing our understanding of what happens to drugs within the body, and has opened a way to safer and more effective drug therapy for patients. With these obvious advantages for the practice of medicine, and with an aura of apparent precision produced by the involvement of mathematics in a clinical area, it is understandable that some prescribers might have allowed themselves to look to the potential of pharmacokinetics with unrealistic hopes. By way of dampening such excessive expectations, the preliminary semiquantitative treatment of the subject which has been developed in this chapter has tried to set some basis for what we hope will be a continuing critical assessment of pharmacokinetic ideas and predictions. The would-be pharmacokineticist should be ever cognisant of the anatomical and physiological factors underlying the fate of drugs in the body, and of the assumptions made in mathematically analysing the time courses of the presence of drugs within the body.

For pharmacokinetics to be thought about and applied in a valid way it is desirable to have an adequate level of knowledge of, and critical scientific insight into:

(1) the mode of action of the drugs in question;
(2) the relevant physiology, biochemistry and anatomy;
(3) the structural and molecular pathology which has led to the use of the drug;
(4) the reliability of the determination of population (and, if available, individual) pharmacokinetic parameters relating to the drug;
(5) the extent of the likely interindividual biological variation in quantitative aspects of the relevant physiology, biochemistry and pharmacokinetics;
(6) the implications of the various pharmacokinetic parameters, the assumptions underlying them and their calculation, and the potential errors inherent in making predictions from pharmacokinetic data, particularly when the predictions relate to quantitative situations beyond those from which the parameters were determined.

As well, it is desirable to have the ability to synthesize these items into unified concepts, and to reason from them.

SOURCES OF PHARMACOKINETIC INFORMATION

Texts on pharmacokinetics

A number of works dealing with pharmacokinetics are available, ranging from introductory accounts to detailed mathematical treatments of the subject. The former include:

Smith, S.E. and Rawlings, M.D. (1973). *Variability in Human Drug Response*. (London: Butterworths)

Eadie, M.J., Tyrer, J.H. and Bochner, F. (1981). *Introduction to Clinical Pharmacology*. (New York: Adis Press)

Benet, L.Z., Massoud, N. and Gambertoglio, L.G. (1984). *Pharmacokinetic Basis for Drug Treatment*. (New York: Raven Press)

Then there are works at an intermediate level of complexity, e.g.

Notari, R.E. (1980). *Biopharmaceutics and Pharmacokinetics. An Introduction.* 3rd Edn. (New York: Dekker)

Rowland, M. and Tozer T.N. (1980). *Clinical Pharmacokinetics. Concepts and Applications* (Philadelphia: Lea and Febiger)

and more advanced mathematical works, e.g.

Wagner, J.G. (1971). *Biopharmaceutics and Relevant Pharmacokinetics.* (Hamilton: Drug Intelligence Publications)

Wagner, J.G. (1975). *Fundamentals of Clinical Pharmacokinetcs.* (Hamilton: Drug Intelligence Publications)

Gibaldi, M. and Perrier, D. (1982). *Pharmacokinetics.* 2nd Edn. (New York: Dekker)

Compendia of pharmacokinetic data

Collections of data concerning the pharmacokinetic properties of a wide range of drugs may be found in:

Pagliaro, L.A. and Benet, L.Z. (1975). *J. Pharmacokin. Biopharmaceut.,* **3**, 333–83

Avery, G. (ed.) (1980). *Drug Treatment.* 2nd Edn. (Sydney: Adis Press)

Gilman, A.G., Goodman, L.S. and Gilman, A. (eds.) (1980): *The Pharmacological Basis of Therapeutics.* 6th Edn. (New York: MacMillan)

Bochner, F., Carruthers, G., Kampmann, J. and Steiner, J. (1983). *Handbook of Clinical Pharmacology* (Boston: Little, Brown & Co.)

Pharmacokinetic research publications and reviews

Original articles dealing with various pharmacokinetic topics and the pharmacokinetic properties of individual drugs appear in many of the common clinical pharmacology journals (and at times elsewhere). However, there is a particular concentration of articles on pharmacokinetics in the following journals:

Journal of Pharmacokinetics and Biopharmaceutics. (Plenum Press)

Clinical Pharmacokinetics. (Adis Press)

The main clinical pharmacology journals include:

British Journal of Clinical Pharmacology

European Journal of Clinical Pharmacology

Clinical Pharmacology and Therapeutics

Arnzmittel-Forschungen (Drug Therapy)

Journal of Clinical Pharmacology

A glossary of pharmacokinetic symbols, which it is hoped will be increasingly adopted internationally, is provided by Rowland, M. and Tucker, G. (1980). *J. Pharmacokin. Biopharmaceut.*, **8**, 497– 507. These symbols are used throughout the present book.

2
Factors determining drug concentrations in the body. The absorption, distribution, metabolism and excretion of drugs

In the brief overview provided in Chapter 1 it was stated that most drugs act after being reversibly bound to receptors, and that the quantitative effect of the drug is then directly related to its concentration in the fluid surrounding the receptors (the 'biophase'). In most instances the concentration of the drug in plasma can be taken as representative of the concentration in the biophase. Therefore the onset, duration and intensity of the pharmacodynamic effect should be reflected in the time course of the concentration of the drug in plasma (Figure 2.1).

A minimum biophase concentration of drug appears to be required for the onset of a particular pharmacodynamic response. For most drugs this concentration is related to a particular concentration of the drug in plasma (the minimum effective concentration, MEC). As long as the drug concentration remains above this minimum level the pharmacological effect is observed. The intensity of the effect increases as the concentration increases, until a maximum response is produced. Beyond this response the effect does not increase even if plasma and biophase drug concentrations increase. The time required for the plasma concentration to reach the minimum effective concentration governs the speed of onset of the particular pharmacodynamic effect under consideration.

To exert their effects, drugs must gain access to, and remain at, their sites of action. Factors influencing the rate and extent of drug absorption from pharmaceutical formulations (drug bioavailability), drug distribution to the site of action and other tissues, and elimination of the drug will, therefore, be important factors in governing the intensity and duration of drug action.

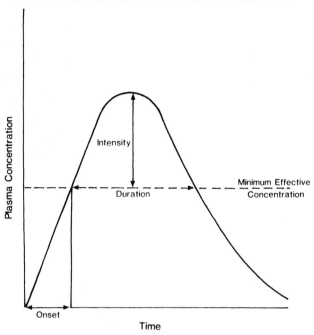

Figure 2.1 Stylized plasma concentration vs. time plot illustrating onset, intensity and duration of a pharmacological effect

A number of factors determine drug concentration in the biophase.

PASSAGE OF DRUGS ACROSS CELL MEMBRANES

After administration, a drug must often traverse several biological membranes in order to reach its receptors. The membranes may be conceptualized as lipid barriers with a protein layer on each side (Figure 2.2). The membranes behave as though they also contain water-filled pores or channels connecting the inside to the outside.

Drugs may cross membranes by several mechanisms which are discussed below.

Passive diffusion

Drug membrane transfer is usually accomplished by passive diffusion. Passive diffusion is the term used to characterize the movement of drug molecules down a concentration gradient without cellular expenditure of energy. This process is neither saturable nor inhibited by other molecules.

The passage of drug molecules across short distances in the body is usually rapid, but passive diffusion may be hindered and sometimes differentially modified by intervening cell membranes. Such membranes may be comparatively simple (e.g. capillary walls, erythrocyte envelope) or complex (e.g. gastrointestinal epithelium) in their molecular arrangement.

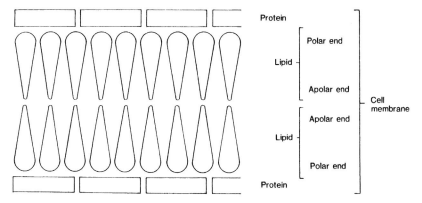

Figure 2.2 An illustration (after Davson, H. and Danielli, J.F. (1952). *Permeability of Natural Membranes.* (New York: Cambridge Univ. Press)) of cell membrane structure. (Reprinted from Eadie, M.J., Tyrer, J.H. and Bochner, F. (1981). *Introduction to Clinical Pharmacology.* p.17; by kind permission of ADIS Press Australasia Pty. Ltd., Sydney)

The rate of passive penetration of the drug through a membrane is governed by Fick's law of diffusion (Equation 2.1), where:

$$\text{Rate of penetration} = \frac{-D.A.K.(C_{out}-C_{in})}{\Delta x} \qquad (2.1)$$

where D is the diffusion coefficient of the drug in the membrane, K is the partition coefficient of the drug between the membrane (lipid) and the aqueous phase on either side of the membrane, A and Δx are the area and thickness of the membrane, respectively, and $(C_{out}-C_{in})$ is the difference between the concentrations of the diffusing drug molecules on the two sides of the membrane.

The partition coefficient, K, is an important determinant of the rate of penetration. When highly lipid soluble drugs (with high values of K) are considered, transfer is very rapid between plasma and tissues, and the rate of intake of such drugs into tissues may be limited only by the blood flow rate. Thus, the entry of general anaesthetics and anaesthetic induction agents into the central nervous system is very rapid.

When a pH difference exists across a membrane, the degree of ionization of the drug molecules on the two sides of the membrane may be an important determinant of the rate of membrane penetration. Ionized molecules possess a high degree of water solubility (i.e. a low K value) and cross membranes much more slowly than their non-ionized counterparts. The latter species are often highly lipid soluble (high K values) and non-polar, and therefore usually have a high rate of membrane penetration.

Consider the case of a weakly basic drug (e.g. ephedrine) and its passage across the membranes of the gastrointestinal epithelia of the stomach and small intestine, respectively. A weak base is poorly absorbed across the gastric mucosa since the normally acidic nature of that environment causes much of the drug to ionize:

$$B + H^+ \leftrightarrow BH^+$$

Conversely, in the more alkaline environment of the small intestine basic drugs may be absorbed quite rapidly. Here the drug molecules are largely unionized and non-polar, and usually are sufficiently lipid soluble to diffuse passively across the epithelial membranes along concentration gradients.

Diffusion through pores

Small polar molecules may diffuse along concentration gradients through water-filled pores in biological membranes. Compounds with molecular weights below 150 (e.g. urea, glycerol) may be transferred across membranes by such processes. Molecules which are too polar, as are many ions, despite having a low molecular size which would permit them to pass through pores, may be so attracted to or repelled by charges carried on the membrane surface or lining the pores that these molecules may not traverse the membrane.

Active transport

Endogenous compounds and some drugs may be transported across membranes against a concentration gradient. This process is termed active transport and requires metabolic energy; it can be inhibited by inhibitors of cellular energy metabolism (e.g. cyanide). Relative selectivity (e.g. stereospecificity), competitive inhibition and saturability serve to characterize active transport processes. Such processes include the 'sodium pump'

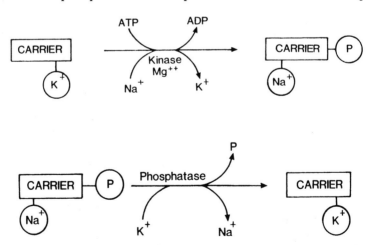

Figure 2.3 (a, b) Active transport as illustrated by the 'sodium-pump'. (Reprinted from Bowman, W.C. and Rand, M.J. (1980). *Textbook of Pharmacology*. 2nd Edn., p.2.8; by kind permission of Blackwell Scientific Publications, Oxford)

(Figure 2.3), the molecular mechanism of which is believed to be as follows.

The terminal phosphate groups from intracellular adenosine triphosphate (ATP) molecules are transferred to carrier molecules in the inner surface of the cell membrane. The phosphorylated carrier, in the presence of magnesium ions, binds Na^+ but not K^+. At the inner surface of the membrane the situation shown in Figure 2.3a exists. The phosphorylated carrier then moves across the membrane to the external surface (Figure 2.3b) where the complex is dephosphorylated and, if potassium ions are present, Na^+ is released and K^+ is bound in its place.

Analogous mechanisms exist for amino acid transfer across cell membranes (e.g. absorption of levodopa from the small intestine). Further examples of active transport of drugs include the secretion of penicillins into the renal tubular lumen and into bile, and the removal of certain anionic drugs from the cerebrospinal fluid into blood by the transport systems of cells in the choroid plexuses.

DRUG ABSORPTION

Absorption from the alimentary tract

Absorption from the stomach and intestine

Oral administration is the most popular route of drug intake. Drugs taken by mouth may be absorbed through the mucous membranes of the buccal mucosa, or the mucosa lining the stomach and/or the small and large intestine.

The efficiency of the oral route of administration for a drug is judged by that drug's bioavailability (see Chapter 5), i.e. the rate and the extent of its entry into the general circulation from the formulation under consideration. Both rate and extent are clinically relevant. The complete absorption of an analgesic or a hypnotic may be of little value to the sufferer if slow absorption results in the minimum effective concentration of the drug not being reached rapidly. In contrast, slow but complete absorption of a drug intended for chronic therapy may be ideal to ensure minimal fluctuations in plasma and biophase drug concentrations, thus producing an even and consistent response.

It is important to remember that a drug must be in solution before it can be absorbed. Many drugs are taken in tablets and capsules, and thus factors such as the solubility, particle size, chemical form, and crystalline characteristics of the drug itself, together with a number of manufacturing variables (compression force used to make tablets, other ingredients in the dosage form, etc.), become important in the release of drug from the formulation and its rate of solution (dissolution) in the fluids of the alimentary tract.

Figure 2.4 is a schematic representation of the steps involved in the release of drug molecules from a solid dosage form. Terms such as disintegration, deaggregation and dissolution are used to describe the steps involved in this process. In particular, such steps become of importance to the clinician when the formulated drug is sparingly soluble in aqueous fluids.

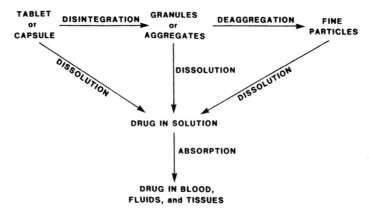

Figure 2.4 Schematic diagram of disintegration, deaggregation and dissolution of a drug from a solid dosage form. (Reprinted from Poole, J.W. (1979). In Blanchard, J., Sawchuk, R.J. and Brodie, B.B. (eds.) *Principles and Perspectives in Drug Bioavailability*. p.76; by kind permission of S. Karger AG, Basel)

In such cases the dissolution rate of the drug may become the rate-limiting step in the process of drug absorption, and in a severe example of slow dissolution a patient may fail to respond to a particular preparation of a drug.

Once a drug is in solution within the fluids of the gastrointestinal tract, a number of factors may operate to influence its absorption. Such factors include absorptive membrane surface area, gastrointestinal motility, environmental pH, local blood flow, the presence of other materials within the gut lumen, gastrointestinal metabolism of the drug, metabolism by gut bacteria, and the effect of disease states.

Area of absorptive membrane – The surface area of the small intestinal mucosa is very large in comparison with the buccal and gastric mucosal surfaces. The absorbing area has been calculated to be of the order of 200 m², taking into consideration the microvilli of the small intestine. The surface area of the stomach is only a small fraction of that of the intestine. Even when the properties of a drug greatly favour gastric over intestinal absorption (i.e. a weakly acidic drug), a large proportion of the ingested dose may still be absorbed from the small intestine because of surface area considerations.

Gastrointestinal motility – The normal stomach acts as a reservoir, and regulates the passage of materials to the duodenum and small intestine. As the absorptive capacity of the small intestine is far larger than that of the stomach, the gastric emptying time is of considerable importance in relation to drug absorption rate. Gastric emptying is particularly critical for formulations which disintegrate or dissolve slowly. Exit of formulations designed to release their contents in the small intestine (enteric coated products) from the stomach may take from 15 min to 7 h; such variability in gastric emptying leads to erratic and unpredictable delivery of whole tablets or capsules into the intestine.

Slowing of gastric emptying rate may be brought about by the presence of food in the stomach, particularly a fatty meal, and by migraine and other disease states. Drugs such as the narcotic-like analgesics, atropine and its anticholinergic congeners, spasmolytics and ganglion blocking agents will produce a similar effect in delaying stomach emptying. Consequently the absorption of co-administered drugs may proceed at a slower rate than for those drugs given alone.

Stimulation of gastric emptying rate may be effected by taking the drug metoclopramide, which may therefore increase the speed of absorption of co-administered medicaments by accelerating their delivery to the absorptive surface of the intestine.

Environmental pH – The effect of environmental pH has been alluded to earlier with reference to the passage of weak bases and weak acids across cell membranes. Weak acids should, in theory, be absorbed from the stomach at its normally acidic pH, while weak bases should be better absorbed from the small intestine. This effect is not of great importance in practice owing to the over-riding influence of the large absorptive surface area of the small intestine relative to the smaller surface area of the stomach. However, the environmental pH of the alimentary tract may affect drug solubility, the rate of dissolution of a drug from a formulation, or drug stability. The effect of pH on the latter is well exemplified by the acid-labile penicillin antibiotics and certain polypeptides (e.g. insulin).

Local blood flow – Apart from its large surface area the small intestine receives the major portion of blood flow to the gastrointestinal tract (some 10% of total cardiac output). This rich blood supply rapidly removes any absorbed drug from the small intestine submucosa, thereby maintaining the drug concentration gradient between lumen and mucosal blood, thus promoting further passage of the drug from the intestinal lumen across the gut mucosa. Gastrointestinal blood supply may be reduced in certain disease states, e.g. congestive cardiac failure. Gastrointestinal absorption of the antiarrhythmic agent quinidine has been shown to be slowed in such circumstances.

Presence of other substances within the lumen – Food and other materials within the gastrointestinal tract may affect drug absorption by binding drugs or forming insoluble complexes with them. Most of the tetracycline antibiotics are poorly absorbed if taken with a meal, or in the presence of antacids, calcium or iron salts with which they chelate. A number of drugs are adsorbed onto finely divided powders (e.g. kaolin), and the absorption of these drugs is thereby reduced; examples of such drugs include lincomycin and promazine. Ion-exchange resins may also sequester some drugs, often reducing the amount of drug available for absorption (e.g. cholestyramine sequestrates digoxin).

Gastrointestinal metabolism – The intestinal mucosa contains a number of enzymes which may metabolically inactivate certain drugs during their passage through the mucosal epithelial cells. Partial inactivation of iso-prenaline, chlorpromazine, oestrogens, levodopa, methyldopa and salicy-lamide has been shown to occur due to this mechanism.

The enzymes of intestinal bacteria are capable of catalysing a number of reactions involving the further metabolism of drugs or drug metabolites. Glucuronide hydrolysis, hydrolysis of amide linkages (e.g. sulphacetamide and sulphathiazole), and glycoside hydrolysis (e.g. anthraquinones) are among these bacterial enzyme-mediated reactions.

Disease states – Congestive cardiac failure (as previously mentioned) may slow the absorption of orally administered drugs, as may pyloric stenosis, which delays gastric emptying. Variable effects on drug absorption have been noted in the different malabsorption states. Other gastrointestinal disorders may affect drug absorption by their influence on gastic emptying time. Emptying rates are significantly lower in patients with gastric ulcers than in normal subjects, while gastric resection may increase gastric emptying rate.

When drugs are absorbed from the stomach or intestine they are carried by the portal circulation to the liver, and after passage through the liver

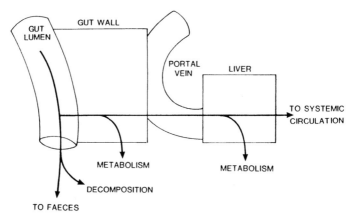

Figure 2.5 First-pass effect; sites of drug loss are indicated by arrows. (Reprinted from Tozer, T.N. (1980). In Blanchard, J., Sawchuk, R.J. and Brodie, B.B. (eds.) *Principles and Perspectives in Drug Bioavailability.* p.127; by kind permission of S. Karger AG, Basel)

enter the systemic circulation (Figure 2.5). Even during their transfer across the intestinal mucosa and their first passage through the liver, some drugs undergo substantial biotransformation. Such drugs include morphine, pe-thidine, pentazocine, lignocaine, acetylsalicylic acid, propranolol, meto-prolol, certain phenothiazines and amitriptyline. This presystemic metabolism, termed the 'first-pass effect', results in an appreciable propor-tion of the absorbed dose not reaching the general circulation intact. Often this presystemic elimination will result in considerable loss of drug effect. As a consequence, a proportionately larger oral dose (as compared with the intravenous or intramuscular dose) may be required to elicit the desired systemic effect.

Absorption after sublingual and buccal administration – Occasionally drugs are given with the intention that they should be absorbed from the buccal mucosa. Due to the relatively thin mucosal surface and its rich blood supply, absorption across the buccal membrane is rapid and has the added advantage of bypassing the portal circulation, thus avoiding first-pass inactivation of drug by the liver.

This route is useful for the administration of glyceryl trinitrate in the treatment of anginal attacks, and has been employed to administer isoprenaline for its bronchodilating action in patients with asthma. Steroids such as testosterone, progesterone and aldosterone may be administered sublingually to avoid hepatic inactivation.

Rectal administration – Administration of drugs by the rectal route, usually in the form of suppositories, may be used to provide either local or systemic effects. The rectum possesses a rich vascular and lymphatic supply, but its mucosa is devoid of villi and has a small surface area relative to its luminal capacity. It has been estimated that approximately two-thirds of a rectally administered drug dose is absorbed directly into the systemic circulation via the inferior and middle haemorrhoidal veins, thus bypassing the portal circulation and avoiding potential first-pass drug inactivation by the liver.

Drug absorption from the rectum is usually slow and erratic. Therefore rectal medication is usually reserved for those clinical situations in which the oral route is unsatisfactory or when only a local mucosal effect is desired. It is particularly useful in children and in patients with severe upper gastrointestinal disturbances and vomiting.

Of recent interest has been the finding that certain drugs which are not normally well absorbed orally (e.g. insulin) may show appreciable absorption from the rectal area in experimental animals.

Absorption through the lungs

Rapid drug absorption occurs by this route if the drug can be delivered into the pulmonary alveoli. The large surface area of the alveoli, the high permeability of the thin alveolar epithelium, and the rich blood supply of the lungs ensures rapid absorption of drugs given in gaseous form by inhalation. Volatile and gaseous anaesthetics are the most important group of drugs given by this route, together with amyl or octyl nitrite for the relief of angina.

Drugs in the form of aerosols or even as solid particles may also be administered by inhalation. In such cases the particle or drop size is critical if the drug is to reach the alveoli. Particle sizes of approximately $0.5-2$ μm diameter are aimed at, since larger particles will impact higher in the respiratory tract and smaller particles will tend to be exhaled again. A careful technique in self-administration of these drugs is also critical or

nt amounts of drug may deposit on the mucosa of the mouth and
be carried by swallowed saliva into the stomach. The main therapeutic
agents given by such inhalation are the bronchodilator drugs such as
salbutamol, isoprenaline and terbutaline. The relatively insoluble cortico-
steroid beclomethasone and sodium cromoglycate (as a powder) are also
given by inhalation for the treatment of asthma. In such cases the therapeutic effect is produced by achieving a high local concentration of drug near
its desired site of action in the bronchiolar wall, with relatively little drug
being absorbed into the circulation.

Absorption through the skin

Medications given by this route are usually intended to act locally to treat
itching or various rashes, to increase the thickness of the keratin layer, to
soften or protect the skin, to provide antisepsis, or to bring antiparasitic
and anti-inflammatory agents to affected areas of skin. The skin epithelial
barrier is thicker and less permeable to drugs than other absorptive surfaces,
and the skin is less well and less consistently perfused with blood. The
partition coefficient of the drug and the nature of the formulation are
critical determinants of therapeutic efficacy in these circumstances. The
rate of drug absorption through the skin is also determined by the site of
application (e.g. thickness and vascularity) and its state (broken, hydrated
or inflammed skin presents a less effective barrier to absorption than
normal skin).

Occasionally, drugs may be sufficiently well absorbed following local
application to produce a systemic effect. Glyceryl trinitrate is slowly
absorbed following cutaneous application and helps prevent angina pectoris
overnight. This route of administration also avoids 'first-pass' metabolism
in the liver.

Intramuscular and subcutaneous administration

Injections are normally given into the muscles of the buttock, the thigh,
or the upper arm, or into the subcutaneous tissue of the arm or thigh. The
injectate spreads between the sheaths of muscle fibres or through the loose
connective tissue of the subcutaneous layer. Both routes of administration
are generally reserved for patients in whom a fairly rapid systemic response
is desired or in whom reliable drug intake is essential, but in whom
intravenous or oral administration is inappropriate or inconvenient. Drug
absorption from intramuscular or subcutaneous sites is usually rapid, but
may be delayed and/or erratic especially when precipitation of the drug
occurs at the injection site (e.g. phenytoin) or when local blood flow is
poor. Absorption of materials following intramuscular or subcutaneous
injection may be deliberately slowed. This may be achieved by adding a
vasoconstrictor to the injection, for example adrenaline may be mixed with
lignocaine for a persisting local anaesthetic effect. Depot preparations
designed to release drug slowly over several hours or days include the
use of water insoluble salts (procaine penicillin), complex suspensions

(protamine zinc insulin), colloids (tetracosactrin), oil bases (fluphenazine enanthate), and implants or drug pellets (testosterone).

Vascular perfusion may limit drug absorption from muscle and subcutaneous tissue. Perfusion varies at different sites. Normally drug absorption is more rapid from the shoulder than from either the thigh or buttock because of differences in blood flow. Rubbing or heating the skin around the injection site may also hasten drug absorption by increasing local blood flow. Subcutaneous blood flow may be reduced in the cold or in states of circulatory failure.

DRUG DISTRIBUTION

Following absorption or intravenous administration, drugs in plasma are transported by the blood, diffuse out of the bloodstream at the level of the capillaries, and are distributed to a variety of locations within the body, including the biophase, the various body fluids and tissue binding sites, and the organs of elimination. The rate of distribution of a drug into a tissue depends on blood flow to the tissue, the permeability of the tissue to the drug, and the partitioning of drug between tissue and plasma. Distribution continues until an equilibrium is established, when the concentrations of drug in plasma water and extracellular water are usually equal. At equilibrium, the extent of distribution depends on the tissue-to-plasma partition ratio and the tissue mass.

Equilibrium develops rapidly for lung, brain, liver and kidney, which are richly perfused; it is established slowly in muscle and fat, which are

Table 2.1 Blood flow to human tissues

Tissue	%Body weight	%Cardiac output	Blood flow ($1 \, kg \, tissue^{-1} \, min^{-1}$)
Adrenals	0.02	1	5.5
Kidneys	0.40	24	4.5
Heart	0.40	4	0.7
Brain	2	15	0.55
Liver	2	5	0.2
Skin	7	5	0.05
Muscle	45	15	0.03
Fat	15	2	0.01

relatively poorly perfused (Table 2.1). Approach to equilibrium for a particular drug may be delayed by poor membrane penetration (e.g. digoxin into cardiac tissue), and by high water solubility of the compound if the tissue in question has a high lipid content (e.g. antibiotics into the central nervous system). Accumulation of thiopentone in muscle and then in fat, following its initial preferential distribution into the central nervous system, may be explained by a combination of poor perfusion of muscle and fat with much greater perfusion of brain plus high lipid solubility of the drug and the brain's high lipid content. The concentration of this anaesthetic agent reaches a peak in adipose tissue some 4–8 h after its administration, at a time when plasma and brain concentrations of the drug have declined greatly, and its anaesthetic effects have largely subsided.

Plasma protein binding

The binding of a drug to plasma proteins may also influence the rate of distribution to tissues. Acidic drugs normally bind to albumin, while basic drugs may bind to albumin, α_1-acid glycoprotein or lipoproteins, and many endogenous compounds bind to globulins.

Binding to plasma proteins is nearly always a reversible process with extremely rapid rates of association and dissociation. Only the unbound (i.e. free) drug in plasma is thought to be capable of diffusing out of the circulation into a tissue. Protein binding acts as a temporary 'store' of a drug, and tends to minimize large fluctuations in the concentration of unbound drug in the body fluids after dosage.

Plasma protein binding is a function of the affinity of the protein for the drug. Only a limited number of protein binding sites is available for complexation, and the extent of binding depends on the concentration of both drug and protein. For a single binding site:

$$D \quad + \quad P \quad \leftrightarrow \quad DP$$

drug   protein   drug–protein
complex

where the association constant K may be expressed in terms of mass law considerations by:

$$K \quad = \quad \frac{[DP]}{[D].[P]} \tag{2.2}$$

If the fraction of the total concentration that is unbound is expressed as fu, then the unbound concentration is $fu.C$ and the bound concentration is $(1-fu).C$. Rearrangement of Equation 2.2 gives:

$$K.[P] \quad = \quad \frac{(1 - fu).C}{fu.C} \quad = \quad \frac{1 - fu}{fu} \tag{2.3}$$

and

$$fu \quad = \quad \frac{1}{1 + K.[P]} \tag{2.4}$$

Thus, the value of fu may be seen to depend on the unbound protein concentration [P] together with the affinity of the protein for the drug, K. The unbound drug concentration is more closely related to the pharmacodynamic activity of the drug than is the total concentration (unbound+bound). Therefore, the value of the fraction of drug that is unbound to plasma proteins is relevant to therapeutics. Approximate values of fu for a number of drugs at normal plasma protein concentrations are shown in Figure 2.6.

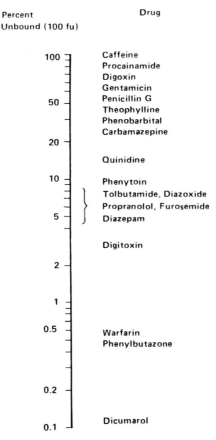

Figure 2.6 Plasma protein binding of a number of therapeutic agents. (Reprinted from Rowland, M. and Tozer, T.N. (1980). *Clinical Pharmacokinetics: Concepts and Applications*. p.43; by kind permission of Lea & Febiger, Philadelphia)

As mentioned in Chapter 1, in clinical practice the unbound drug concentration is measured only occasionally because the methods available for doing so are often slow and tedious. A higher degree of analytical sensitivity is also required to quantitate the unbound concentration for a drug which is highly protein bound. Whole blood concentrations of a drug are sometimes to be preferred over the plasma concentration for assessing the distribution of drug into and its elimination from tissues, since it is drug in whole blood and not just that in plasma which is delivered to tissues.

In most instances the percentage of unbound drug in plasma remains reasonably constant over the range of drug concentrations in plasma associated with usual dosage regimens. However, non-linear plasma protein binding may sometimes occur with basic drugs at clinical dosage (e.g. disopyramide). Displacement of bound drug from plasma proteins can occur when the same binding sites are competed for by displacing agents. Such behaviour is clinically relevant only when the displaced drug has a small apparent volume of distribution and is present in high concentration (e.g. the sulphonamides, salicylate and phenylbutazone).

Some variability has been noted in plasma protein binding capacity in disease states. A decrease in the apparent affinity of the proteins for drugs has been observed in uraemia, and the concentration of binding proteins may be altered, e.g. albumin is decreased in chronic liver disease, and α_1-acid glycoprotein increased in stress conditions.

Tissue binding

The fraction of drug in the body located in the plasma is also dependent

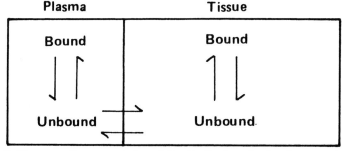

Figure 2.7 Diagrammatic representation of the distribution of a drug between plasma and tissues. (Reprinted from Rowland, M. and Tozer, T.N. (1980). *Clinical Pharmacokinetics: Concepts and Applications*. p.44; by kind permission of Lea & Febiger, Philadelphia)

on drug binding to tissue components (Figure 2.7). The affinity of a tissue for a drug may be the result of its binding to tissue proteins and to nucleic acids and, in the case of adipose tissue, dissolution in fat. Unlike plasma binding, tissue binding of a drug cannot be measured directly. Handling of a tissue (which would be necessary for the measurement) tends to result in its disruption and loss of integrity. Further, the extent of drug binding may vary from tissue to tissue, and, within a tissue, from one component to another.

Sequestration of drugs by tissues and selected tissue components is illustrated by the data in Table 2.2.

Apparent volume of distribution

The amount of a drug in the body can never be measured directly in man. Observations can be made on the concentration of drug in plasma, and such information is used to calculate the apparent volume of distribution of the drug. This parameter is defined as the volume of fluid the drug would occupy if the total amount of drug in the body were at the same concentration as is present in plasma, i.e.:

$$\text{Volume of distribution} = \frac{\text{Amount in body}}{\text{Plasma drug concentration}}$$

Table 2.2 Sequestration of drugs by tissue and tissue constituents

Drug	Tissue	Tissue component
Griseofulvin	Hair, nails, skin	Keratin
Chloroquine	Skin, eye	Melanin
Mepacrine	Liver, pancreas, leukocytes	Nucleic acids
Sulphasalazine	?	Collagen
Thiopentone, ether, insecticides	Adipose tissues	Fat
Tetracyclines	Growing bones and teeth	Calcium
Iodine	Thyroid	

The apparent volume of distribution is a direct but somewhat imperfect measure of the extent of a drug's distribution. Its value rarely, however, corresponds to an actual physiological volume. A drug may be distributed to various tissues and fluids of the body, and may not achieve the same concentrations in each of these components as in plasma. The extent of drug binding to tissue components may be so great that the apparent volume of distribution works out to be many times the total physical body volume because the drug's concentration in tissues is higher than in plasma. Values of the apparent volume of distribution for several drugs are shown in Figure 2.8. For a more detailed analysis of the pharmacokinetic concept of distribution volumes for a drug the reader is referred to Chapter 5.

Blood–brain barrier

The existence in the central nervous system of a mechanism capable of excluding from the neural parenchyma many substances carried in the bloodstream has been recognized for many years. This mechanism has been termed 'the blood–brain barrier'. The barrier is not absolute and represents a quantitative rather than a qualitative difference in capillary permeability as compared with other tissues. The footplates of astrocytes of the central nervous system are closely applied to the capillary basement membrane, and a substance passing from the capillary lumen to the interstitial fluid surrounding the neurons must penetrate both the membranes of the capillary endothelium and the astrocyte footplates. However, the main component in the blood–brain barrier effect appears to be the tight intercellular junctions of the cerebral vascular endothelium. The blood–brain barrier effect is lacking in a few specialized regions of the brain, e.g. the vomiting centre in the medulla, the anterior perforated substance, parts of the hypothalamus and the pineal body.

Strongly protein bound drugs are largely excluded by this barrier with some exceptions (e.g. diazepam), as are poorly fat soluble drugs. In general

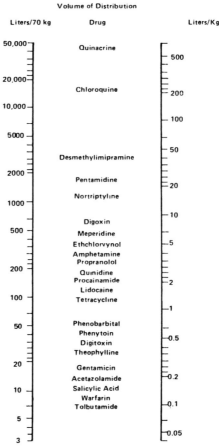

Figure 2.8 The apparent distribution volume of a number of drugs. (Reprinted from Rowland, M. and Tozer, T.N. (1980). *Clinical Pharmacokinetics: Concepts and Applications*. p.40; by kind permission of Lea & Febiger, Philadelphia)

there is a good correlation between rate of penetration into the brain and lipid solubility. The more lipid soluble substances pass through the barrier more easily.

Penetration of drugs into the cerebrospinal fluid is proportional to the concentration of unbound drug in plasma, and drug concentrations in CSF and plasma water are often virtually identical. However, active extrusion of acidic drugs from the CSF may occur at the level of the choroid plexus (e.g. various penicillin antibiotics) and may reduce CSF drug concentrations below plasma concentrations of unbound substance for these drugs.

DRUG ELIMINATION

Drug biotransformation (metabolism), mainly by the liver, and renal excretion are the major routes of drug elimination (i.e. clearance) from the body. Less important routes include excretion via the biliary tract, via the lungs, and in sweat and in other secretions, or in body fluids that are lost in pathological states.

Hepatic biotransformation

Generally, the biotransformation of a drug decreases its lipid solubility by converting it into a more polar and therefore more water soluble metabolite, facilitating the subsequent renal excretion of this metabolite. Often these polar drug metabolites are less active than the parent drug, or are inactive pharmacologically. This change in pharmacodynamic property may be brought about by the decreased receptor activation capacity of the metabolite, or by a decreased ability of the metabolite to cross cell membranes to reach receptors.

Drug biotransformation often occurs in two stages, or 'phases':

(1)   an initial reaction (Phase I) in which there is a change in the drug molecule itself, for example, oxidation, reduction or hydrolysis. In such reactions the metabolites produced may still be pharmacologically active.

(2)   a conjugation reaction (Phase II) which may be subsequent to (1) in which a conjugate is formed between a drug (or a drug metabolite produced in a Phase I reaction) and an endogenous molecule.

The main site of drug biotransformation is the liver. Many drugs are substrates for the microsomal enzymes of the hepatocyte. The kidney, lung, intestinal mucosa, plasma and nervous tissue also contain important drug metabolizing enzymes.

Phase I reactions – These reactions (oxidations, reductions, or hydrolyses) result in the introduction or uncovering of polar groups in the drug molecule. The metabolizing enzymes necessary for nearly all the oxidations are known as the mixed function oxidases (mono-oxygenases), and require the presence of the reduced form of nicotinamide-adenine dinucleotide phosphate (NADPH), molecular oxygen, and cytochrome P_{450}. They are

Table 2.3 Common Phase I metabolic reactions

Oxidations	Hydrolysis	Reductions
Hydroxylation	Deamidation	Aldehyde reduction
Dealkylation	De-esterification	Azoreduction
Oxide formation		Nitroreduction
Dehalogenation		
Alcohol oxidation		
Desulphuration		
Aldehyde oxidation		

located mainly in the microsomal fraction of the cell. Table 2.3 indicates the more common Phase I reactions.

Phase II reactions – Phase II reactions involve the coupling of the original drug molecule or metabolite to an organic acid (glucuronic acid, sulphate, mercapturic acid) or other group (acylation, acetylation, *O*-methylation, glycine conjugation). These reactions produce compounds which are normally pharmacologically inactive as well as being highly water soluble. Phase II reactions are also often the rate-limiting steps in overall drug biotransformation.

Factors affecting drug biotransformation

Hepatic blood flow and intrinsic metabolizing capacity of the liver – See Chapter 5 for a discussion of these factors, and the pharmacokinetic concept of hepatic extraction and its influence on drug clearance.

Age – It would appear that it takes some weeks after birth for a number of the drug metabolizing enzyme systems to achieve the functioning capacities seen in childhood. Different enzyme systems mature at different times. Both glucuronide formation and mixed function oxidations are relatively underdeveloped in the neonate, as compared with older children and adults. Plasma esterase activity may also be low in the neonate, while the capacities to form glycine and sulphate conjugates may approximate those of the adult.

In older children a period of more rapid biotransformation may occur

Table 2.4 Some pharmacokinetic properties of diazepam in different age groups (from Mandelli, M., Tognoni, G. and Garattini, S. (1978). Clinical pharmacokinetics of diazepam. *Clin. Pharmacokin.*, **3**, 72–91)

Age	Halflife* (h)	Clearance* (ml kg^{-1} h^{-1})
Premature infants (28–34 weeks)	75±37	27.49±8.53
Newborn (1–2 days)	31±2.2	–
Children (4–8 years)	18±3	102.10±9.72
Adults	51±7	16.73±2.19

*The concepts of halflife and clearance are discussed in Chapter 5

as compared with the adult (Table 2.4). In such circumstances it may be necessary to use a higher dose of a drug than in the adult (on a body weight basis) to attain the same pharmacodynamic effect. Examples of drugs whose dosage may need to be higher relative to body weight in children include phenytoin and theophylline.

At the other extreme of the age spectrum, the elderly patient, there may be a reduction in drug metabolizing capacity probably as a result of diminished liver mass and hepatic blood flow. Some evidence of an age-related selective effect on biotransformation exists, and it would appear that Phase I reactions are normally decreased with ageing while Phase II processes may be unaffected. Studies with the benzodiazepine class of compounds confirm this finding in relation to chlordiazepoxide, diazepam and desmethyldiazepam which undergo Phase I reactions. Oxazepam, lorazepam and temazepam are principally metabolized by conjugation, and do not show the effect to the same extent.

Sex – There are examples of different rates of biotransformation between the sexes, but in general this factor has not been shown to be an important source of variation and may have little clinical significance.

Pregnancy – Drug biotransformation may be altered during pregnancy. Most evidence suggests that an increase in drug metabolizing capacity occurs in pregnant women, and drug dosage requirements may need to be adjusted upwards. The anticonvulsants phenytoin and phenobarbitone show such an increased elimination in pregnancy.

Genetic factors – A number of well defined examples of genetically determined variability in the capacity to biotransform drugs is known. Perhaps the most studied example is that of drug acetylation. On the basis of their capacity to acetylate drugs, populations may be divided into two

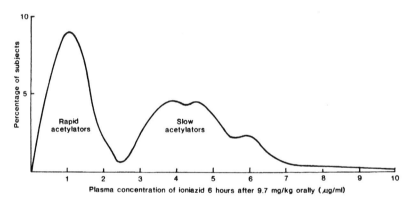

Figure 2.9 Distribution of rapid and slow acetylators of isoniazid in a group of subjects from Caucasian families (data from Evans, D.A.P., Manley, K.A. and Kusick, V.C. (1960). *Br. Med. J.*, **2**, 485–491). (Reprinted from Bowman, W.C. and Rand, M. (1980). *Textbook of Pharmacology*. 2nd Edn. p.4.29; by kind permission of Blackwell Scientific Publications, Oxford)

groups,'slow' and 'fast' acetylators (Figure 2.9). The relevant metabolizing enzyme is a hepatic *N*-acetylase which displays genetic polymorphism. The difference between the phenotypes is due to differences in the amount rather than the nature of the enzyme. Acetylation is an important metabolic pathway in the elimination of isoniazid, hydrallazine, sulphamethazine, nitrazepam, procainamide and phenelzine. Toxicity from these drugs is more likely to occur in slow than in fast acetylators (e.g. the systemic lupus erythematosus syndrome with hydrallazine). However, hepatic toxicity from isoniazid has been associated with rapid acetylation capacity.

A rare genetically determined deficiency in the enzyme pseudocholinesterase may occur in man. The enzyme catalyses the hydrolysis of certain choline esters including the muscle relaxant succinylcholine. Deficiency of this enzyme may cause prolonged apnoea in patients given succinylcholine during surgery.

More recently, evidence has been accumulating on genetic variations in the biotransformation of drugs by the mixed function oxidase system of the liver. Initially such data were limited to the antihypertensive agent debrisoquin, but several more important drug examples have now been noted.

Disease – Hepatic disease may or may not be associated with a reduced capacity to biotransform drugs. The reserve metabolic capacity of the liver is so great that no observable decrease in biotransformation is noted until liver function becomes very severely affected, as in advanced hepatic cirrhosis or hepatic failure. Table 2.5 illustrates the variation that exists in studies of drug elimination in liver disease.

Drug dosage may need to be adjusted in patients with hepatic function impairment. An adjustment in dosage is particularly warranted when the usual regimen might result in drug accumulating to toxic levels as a result of a decrease in its elimination.

At present no clearcut relationship exists between the pharmacokinetic parameters of a drug, especially hepatic clearance, and any appropriate conventional laboratory measure of hepatic function. Thus dosage adjustment in patients with liver disease remains arbitrary and dependent on clinical acumen and plasma drug concentration measurement.

Enzyme induction – The activity of hepatic microsomal enzyme systems can be increased by exposure to a number of substrates (Table 2.6). The most active inducing agents include the barbiturates (in particular, phenobarbitone), rifampicin, and the polycyclic aromatic hydrocarbons.

The class of compound exemplified by phenobarbitone produces an increase in microsomal enzyme activity accompanied by an increase in size and weight of the liver, at least in experimental animals. Hepatic microsomal protein, lipid and cytochrome P_{450} contents are increased. Phenobarbitone induction in animals begins within 1 day of exposure to the drug, and increases over a few days; it diminishes again over 1–3 weeks after the phenobarbitone is discontinued.

Induction of the polycyclic aromatic hydrocarbon type differs from that produced by other substrates in a number of ways, the most important being that its maximal effect occurs very rapidly (24 h or less), while that of the phenobarbitone type drugs takes several days. Chronic administration of phenobarbitone reduces the effectiveness of the coumarin anticoagulants (dicoumarol, warfarin), and the dose of anticoagulant may need to be increased to produce the desired effect on coagulation. Discontinuation

Table 2.5 Changes in total clearance (CL) and elimination halflife ($t_{\frac{1}{2}}$) of some drugs in liver disease

Drug	Disease	Parameter	
		CL	$t_{\frac{1}{2}}$
Ampicillin	Cirrhosis	↓	↑
Amylobarbitone	Cirrhosis	↓	↑
Chloramphenicol	Cirrhosis	★	↑
Diazepam	Cirrhosis	↓	↑
Isoniazid	Cirrhosis	★	↑
Lignocaine	Cirrhosis	↓	↑
Oxazepam	Cirrhosis	⟷	⟷
Pancuronium	Cirrhosis	↓	↑
Pethidine	Cirrhosis	↓	↑
Phenobarbitone	Cirrhosis	★	↑
Phenylbutazone	Cirrhosis	★	↑
Tolbutamide	Cirrhosis	⟷	⟷
Diazepam	Acute viral hepatitis	↓	↑
Lignocaine	Acute viral hepatitis	⟷	⟷
Pethidine	Acute viral hepatitis	↓	↑
Phenobarbitone	Acute viral hepatitis	★	⟷
Phenylbutazone	Acute viral hepatitis	★	⟷
Phenytoin	Acute viral hepatitis	⟷	⟷
Warfarin	Acute viral hepatitis	⟷	⟷
Diazepam	Chronic hepatitis	↓	↑
Pancuronium	Chronic biliary obstruction	↓	↑

⟷ = Parameter unchanged; ↑ = increased; ↓ = decreased; ★ = only halflife measured

of the inducing agent would also necessitate careful monitoring of the prothrombin time, while anticoagulant dosage is readjusted downward over a number of days.

The induction by drugs of hepatic microsomal enzymes that catalyse their own metabolism ('auto-induction') is believed to play a part in the development of apparent tolerance to some sedatives and hypnotics.

Enzyme inhibition – Many substrates for microsomal enzymes may act as competitive antagonists to the mono-oxygenase system. Some substrates

Table 2.6 Inducers of liver microsomal enzyme activities

Alkaloids	Nicotine, cotinine
Analgesics	Phenazone
Anti-inflammatory agents	Phenylbutazone
Anticoagulants	Coumarins
Anticonvulsants	Carbamazepine, methoin, phenytoin, primidone
Antifungals	Clotrimazole, griseofulvin
Antihistamines	Chlorcyclizine, cyclizine, diphenhydramine
Antilipidaemics	Halofenate
Muscle relaxants	Carisoprodol, mephenesin, orphenadrine
Diuretics	Spironolactone
Hypoglycaemics	Tolbutamide
Narcotics	Pethidine
Sedative hypnotics	Barbiturates, chloral hydrate, chlordiazepoxide, dichloralphenazone, glutethimide, methaqualone, meprobamate
Steroids	Adrenocorticoids, androgens, progestogens
Uricosurics	Probenecid
Psychotropics	Chlorpromazine, imipramine, promazine, fluopromazine
Polycyclic hydrocarbons	3-methylcholanthrene, 3-4 benzpyrene
Insecticides	Aldrin, dieldrin, eldrin, lindane, chlordane, DDT, etc.
Miscellaneous	Cigarette smoking, diet, ethanol
Industrial chemicals	Benzene, polychlorinated biphenyls (PCBs)

may yield end products that produce a non-competitive inhibition by disruption of components of the microsomal enzyme system. These substrates act as enzyme inhibitors and may decrease the rate of biotransformation of various co-administered drugs. Examples of such substances include disulfiram and cimetidine. Inhibition of the mitochondrial enzyme, monoamine oxidase (MAO), is sometimes used therapeutically to prolong the action of endogenous amines, e.g. in treating depression or obsessional states. Monoamine oxidase inhibitors are potent (often irreversible) inhibitors of monoamine oxidase, and interactions of these drugs with other agents (e.g. pressor amines) that are metabolized by monoamine oxidases are of considerable clinical significance: some are potentially lethal, and others are responsible for an increase in the severity of toxicity and unwanted side-effects of the co-administered drug.

Drug excretion

Renal excretion

The three mechanisms involved in the urinary excretion of drugs are glomerular filtration, tubular secretion and tubular reabsorption (Figure 2.10).

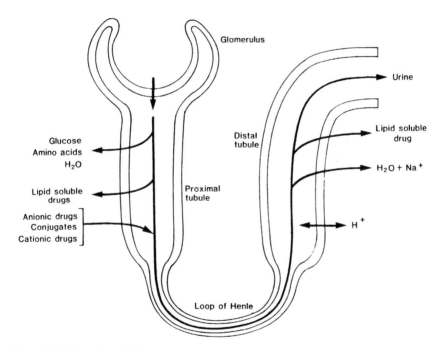

Figure 2.10 Functions of different parts of the nephron. (Reprinted from Eadie, M.J., Tyrer, J.H. and Bochner, F. (1981). *Introduction to Clinical Pharmacology.* p.77; by kind permission of ADIS Press Australasia Pty. Ltd., Sydney)

Glomerular filtration – Renal blood flow is of the order of 1.2–1.5 l/min (renal plasma flow 0.6–0.8 l/min), and of this flow volume about 10% is filtered at the glomerulus into the urine. Only drug in plasma water is filtered, due to the inability of the glomerulus to filter molecules as large as albumin, or larger. Thus drug bound to macromolecules or erythrocytes is unable to pass across the glomerular membranes. The glomerular filtrate contains the drug at a concentration identical to that in plasma water. The rate at which plasma water is filtered (approx. 125 ml/min) is the glomerular filtration rate (GFR). GFR is normally estimated with reference to the (administered) inulin clearance, though clearance of endogenous creatinine is sometimes used as a measure of glomerular filtration.

Tubular secretion – In the epithelium of the proximal convoluted tubule there are active transport mechanisms for the excretion of strong acids and bases from plasma water into urine. Secretion can sometimes be so extensive that nearly all of the drug in blood is removed, whether or not it is bound to plasma proteins or red blood cells. Tubular secretory capacity (active transport maximum) of the kidneys may be assessed with reference to one such compound, *p*-aminohippuric acid, whose clearance approximates 480 ml/min. Competitive inhibition of these active transport processes may occur as evidenced by the effect of probenecid, a competitive inhibitor of active transport of anions (penicillins, cephalosporins). Evidence now exists for the competitive inhibition of cation transport by drugs of basic character (e.g. cimetidine and procainamide).

In some instances the active transport functions overall in a reverse direction (e.g. for uric acid). That is, uric acid undergoes net reabsorption from the tubular lumen.

Tubular reabsorption – Tubular reabsorption varies from being almost absent to being virtually complete for different drugs. Active reabsorption occurs for many endogenous compounds, including vitamins, electrolytes, glucose and amino acids. For many drugs, however, reabsorption is a passive process. The degree of reabsorption depends on the physical properties of the drug. Factors such as the drug's lipid solubility, state of ionization, and molecular weight may be determinants of the extent of its tubular reabsorption. Tubular membranes act as a barrier to water-soluble and ionized molecules. Thus while lipid soluble compounds tend to be extensively reabsorbed, polar molecules do not. Reabsorption also depends on physiological factors such as the rate of urine flow and urinary pH (which influences the extent of drug ionization). The body adjusts urine pH in the distal renal tubules to preserve extracellular fluid H^+ concentration within narrow limits. This urine pH adjustment alters the extent of drug ionization, and hence the amount of drug resorption, while drugs pass in the urine down the distal renal tubules.

When the urine is made more acid, the degree of ionization of basic drugs is increased and their reabsorption is consequently depressed, since only the unionized species resorbs. Conversely, the ionization of acidic drugs is decreased and their reabsorption is enhanced. For an alkaline urine the opposite is true. This finding has found clinical application in producing a forced diuresis of salicylate following overdosage, by alkalinizing the urine with sodium bicarbonate.

Renal clearance – The appearance of a drug in urine is the net result of filtration, secretion and reabsorption. The rate of excretion is, therefore:

$$\text{Rate of excretion} \quad = \quad \text{Rate of filtration}$$
$$+ \quad \text{Rate of secretion}$$
$$- \quad \text{Rate of reabsorption}$$

When the rate of excretion of a drug is directly proportional to its plasma concentration (C) then:

$$\text{Rate of excretion} \quad = \quad CL_R.C$$

where CL_R is the renal clearance, and is equal to the volume (ml) of plasma which in theory would have been completely cleared of the drug by the kidney per minute. The concept of clearance is discussed further in Chapter 5. The classical calculation of renal clearance is by the use of the following equation:

$$\text{Renal clearance} \quad = \quad \frac{\text{Concentration in urine } (\mu g/ml) \ast \text{Rate of urine formation (ml/min)}}{\text{Concentration in plasma } (\mu g/ml)}$$

Renal clearance of a drug may be expressed as a ratio to the GFR by:

$$\text{Clearance ratio} \quad = \quad \frac{\text{Renal clearance}}{\text{GFR}}$$

A ratio greater than unity implies the occurrence of tubular excretion: thus the clearance ratio of benzylpenicillin is 5.2. A clearance of less than unity implies the occurrence of tubular reabsorption: for ethanol, for example, the ratio is about 0.008. However, it should be remembered that the one drug may undergo both tubular secretion and tubular reabsorption. Thus a clearance ratio greater than 1 simply allows the inference that net tubular secretion has occurred, but not that there was no tubular reabsorption.

For a more detailed discussion of the quantitative aspects of renal excretion, including the significance of renal disease, the reader is referred to Chapters 3 and 5.

Other routes of drug excretion

Biliary excretion – A number of drugs may be actively secreted into the intestine via the bile. There appear to be three main transport systems: one each for acids, bases and non-ionized molecules.

Molecular size appears to be an important determinant of the extent of biliary excretion of a drug, since only compounds with molecular weights greater than 350 are extensively excreted in bile. Examples of drugs actively secreted into bile include ampicillin, tetracycline, rifampicin, colchicine, sulindac, indomethacin, tubocurarine, cardiac glycosides, and a number of steroids (testosterone, oestradiol, norethynodrel). Biliary secretion of drug metabolites and their conjugates may also be quite extensive.

The drug and/or its metabolites entering the intestine from the bile may be excreted from the body in the faeces. However, drug or drug metabolite reabsorption from the intestine may also occur. Drug conjugates may be hydrolysed in the gut, with liberation of the active drug, thus permitting an enterohepatic shunt or recycling of the drug. The effect of the shunt is to increase the persistence of the drug in the body, and perhaps thereby to prolong its duration of action. Such enterohepatic shunts have been noted for phenolphthalein, chloramphenicol and stilboestrol. These drugs are converted to glucuronides by hepatic metabolism and are secreted as the conjugates into the bile. In the intestine, bacterial enzyme hydrolysis of the glucuronides occurs to liberate the unconjugated drug which may then be reabsorbed.

Excretion in saliva, sweat, tears, milk and expired air – Saliva, sweat and tears are very minor routes of drug excretion, and milk is a route of excretion only in the special circumstances of lactation. Drugs pass into these secretions principally by passive diffusion of the unionized form. The rate and extent of such transport is determined by the usual factors (see above).

Excretion of drugs into the milk of nursing mothers may be of concern because of the possibility of adverse reactions in the breast-fed infant. However, maternal drug intake in therapeutic dosage usually will not result in the infant receiving more than about 8% of the administered dose in breast milk, an amount unlikely to have any significant clinical consequences for most drugs. When the mother is overdosed, or is treated with potentially toxic drugs (e.g. cytotoxic agents) or with drugs which affect thyroid function (e.g. propylthiouracil, iodides), there may be a distinct possibility of the infant being adversely affected.

Excretion of drugs in the expired air from the lungs readily occurs with volatile lipid soluble substances, such as ethyl alcohol and paraldehyde, but is of importance only in the excretion of the volatile anaesthetic agents. Monitoring of radioactivity in the expired air has been used as an index of hepatic drug metabolizing capacity for substances which are metabolized to CO_2, e.g. the [^{14}C]aminopyrine breath test.

3
Derivation of pharmacokinetic parameters

There are many biological and physicochemical processes which influence drug disposition. Diffusion, enzyme-mediated metabolic reactions, and liquid flow rates are but a few. It could be anticipated that the mathematical formulae needed to describe all these processes in combination would be quite complex; many parameters would be required to describe protein binding, tissue binding, metabolic processes, and drug disposition in detail. In many cases, however, the potentially complicated situation arising from these processes can be simplified because, relative to the concentration of drug or the amount of drug in the body tissues, these processes are of large magnitude and are therefore relatively constant in rate throughout the period of drug exposure. For example, even though enzyme kinetics are often quite complex, if there is more than enough enzyme present to metabolize the drug present at any given time, then the rate of the enzyme-mediated reaction will depend only on the drug concentration for that drug exposure. Changes in enzyme concentration would naturally alter the drug kinetics, but during a particular drug exposure it is often possible to treat the enzyme concentration and activity as a constant. For these reasons, a highly simplified approach is often sufficient to mathematically describe the absorption, distribution, metabolism and excretion of many drugs at the dosages used in man. The time course of plasma and urine concentrations of drug and metabolite determined after the administration of many drugs can be satisfactorily explained by assuming that the body behaves as a single well-mixed compartment in relation to the drug dose, with first order transfer or disposition processes. In the case of other drugs, postulating two or more body compartments may be required to mathematically describe the data collected. In this chapter we will describe mathematically these different compartmental models, both with equations and graphically.

ONE-COMPARTMENT MODELS

In the one-compartment model it is assumed that drug concentrations throughout the body are in rapid equilibrium during the period of drug exposure. This does not mean that drug concentrations are necessarily equal in all tissues, but implies that the distribution processes are very rapid. The body can then be represented by a single compartment (Figure

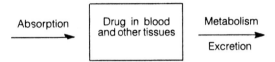

Figure 3.1 Diagram of the one-compartment model showing absorption and the elimination processes, metabolism and excretion

3.1) with an apparent volume (of distribution), V. Also included in this scheme are absorption, metabolism and excretion processes.

The conceptual model can be further defined by considering the processes of absorption and elimination (both metabolism and excretion) individually. The absorption process depends on the route of administration. If the drug is given by rapid intravenous (i.v.) injection there is no absorption process to consider. If we assume rapid mixing of the drug in the blood as well as fast distribution of the drug in the body, a rapid i.v. injection can be represented as if we have instantaneously dissolved the drug in the body. Alternatively, the drug may be given as an i.v. infusion at a constant rate. This rate is a *zero order rate process* because it is not dependent on the concentration or amount of drug remaining to be infused (Equation 3.1).

$$\text{Rate} \quad = \quad \text{constant} \tag{3.1}$$

The infusion process is then the 'absorption' step which will cause an increase in the amount and concentration of drug in the body. If a drug is given by a route other than the intravenous, the drug must be absorbed across one or more biological membranes before it can enter the general circulation. Drugs given orally must be absorbed across the linings of the gastrointestinal tract; drugs given by intramuscular or subcutaneous injection must diffuse through tissues and across the lining of blood capillaries. In many cases the absorption of a drug from the site of administration to the body compartment can be described by a single *first order process*. A rate process is of first order when the rate of the process is proportional to the amount of substance remaining to undergo the process (Equation 3.2).

$$\text{Rate of absorption} = \quad \text{constant} \quad \times \quad \begin{array}{l}\text{amount remaining}\\\text{to be absorbed}\end{array} \tag{3.2}$$

Radioactive decay is an example of a first order process. The rate of decay is proportional to the amount of material remaining. Occasionally drug absorption may be better described by a series of first order steps or even by zero order kinetics, much like an i.v. infusion.

Although the underlying mechanisms involved in drug metabolism and excretion may be quite varied and complex, these processes can often be adequately described mathematically by first order kinetics. Drug metabolism is almost always enzyme mediated. One would expect it to be described by Michaelis–Menten kinetics, but at low drug (substrate) concentration relative to the K_m value first order kinetics can describe the Michaelis–Menten process adequately. Drug concentrations in human therapeutics are usually low relative to enzyme capacity. Therefore, most metabolic processes can be described by first order kinetics (apparent first order kinetics). Also, most excretion pathways involve passive filtration or diffusion and therefore they too can be described by first order kinetics.

Single rapid i.v. injections

The simplest pharmacokinetic model is the one-compartment model with a single first order elimination step. If the drug is administered as a rapid i.v. injection the absorption process can be ignored. This model is shown in Figure 3.2.

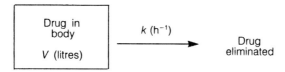

Figure 3.2 Diagram of the one-compartment model showing the pharmacokinetic parameters V and k

We can easily calculate the anticipated initial plasma concentration by dividing the dose administered by the apparent volume of distribution.

$$C(0) = \text{DOSE}/V \tag{3.3}$$

The next step is to describe the equation for the rate of drug elimination. If the elimination step is first order, the rate of elimination is proportional to the concentration of drug in the body. Therefore, dC/dt, the rate of change of C, can be calculated using Equation 3.4:

$$dC/dt = - k.C \tag{3.4}$$

where k is the elimination rate constant, i.e. the fraction of drug in the body eliminated per unit time (e.g. $0.1\ h^{-1}$).

The elimination rate constant can be used to describe how quickly a drug is eliminated. Equation 3.4 can be integrated to yield an equation for C at any time (t) after a rapid i.v. injection.

$$C = C(0).e^{-k.t} \tag{3.5}$$

or

$$C = (\text{DOSE}/V) .e^{-k.t} \tag{3.6}$$
since $C(0) = \text{DOSE}/V$.

Equation 3.6 can be used to calculate the plasma concentration at any time after a single rapid i.v. injection of a drug. A typical plasma

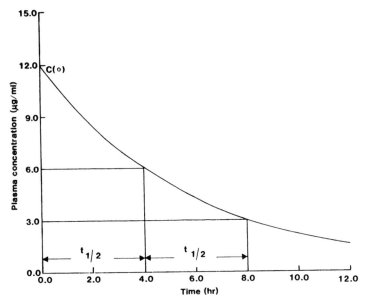

Figure 3.3 Linear plot of plasma concentration vs. time after a single i.v. bolus dose. Illustrated is the drop in plasma concentration from $C(0)$ to $C(0)/2$ and $C(0)/4$ in one and two halflives

concentration vs. time curve is shown in Figure 3.3. The curve in this figure was calculated using a dose of 300 mg, a V of 25 l, and a k of 0.17 h^{-1} (or $t_{\frac{1}{2}}$ of 4 h, see below).

Another parameter commonly used to describe the elimination of a drug is the elimination (or biological) halflife, $t_{\frac{1}{2}}$. When the elimination process follows first order kinetics the halflife will be independent of the concentration. For example, in Figure 3.3 the plasma concentration will fall from $C(0)$ to $C(0)/2$ in the same time that it takes to drop from $C(0)/2$ to $C(0)/4$. This time, $t_{\frac{1}{2}}$, can be calculated from Equation 3.5 if we know k.

$$C(0)/2 = C(0).e^{-k.t_{\frac{1}{2}}}$$

Taking the logarithm (base e) of both sides and rearranging gives:

$$\begin{aligned} t_{\frac{1}{2}} &= \ln(2)/k \\ &= 0.693/k \end{aligned} \tag{3.7}$$

One final parameter can be defined before considering other routes of drug administration. This parameter is the total body clearance (CL) or plasma clearance, which can be described in terms of the volume of plasma that is cleared of drug per unit time. For example, if the only method of drug elimination is by liver metabolism and if the drug is so efficiently metabolized by the liver that all the drug in plasma which reaches the liver is converted to metabolites, then the total body clearance will be equal to the plasma flow to the liver per unit time. In this situation the total volume of plasma which reaches the liver will be cleared of drug. The total body clearance can be calculated using Equation 3.8.

$$CL = k.V \qquad (3.8)$$

In effect, the situation is as if part of the drug's apparent volume of distribution is completely cleared of drug in each unit of time, with the drug concentration remaining unaltered in the remainder of the volume.

Single i.v. infusion

For some drugs a rapid i.v. dose may produce initial toxic plasma concentrations. For this or other reasons prolonged intravenous administration may be preferred. In these cases an i.v. infusion may be used to administer the drug. Instead of a single i.v. dose, a suitable constant rate of drug infusion and duration of infusion is chosen. During the infusion administration the model in Figure 3.4 is appropriate.

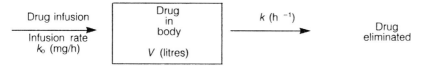

Figure 3.4   Diagram of the one-compartment model showing drug infusion and drug elimination

The rate of change of plasma concentration is now governed by two rate processes, an input process (k_o/V) and an output process $(k.C)$, as shown in Equation 3.9.

$$dC/dt = \text{Rate in} - \text{Rate out}$$
$$= k_o/V - k.C \qquad (3.9)$$

This equation can be integrated to give an equation for the plasma concentration at any time during an infusion, Equation 3.10.

$$C = \frac{k_o}{V.k} . [1 - e^{-k.t}] \qquad (3.10)$$

The resulting plasma concentration vs. time curve is illustrated in Figure 3.5.

If the infusion is continued indefinitely the plasma concentration will increase until the rate of elimination (which increases as drug concentration increases) becomes equal to the rate of infusion. At this point a steady

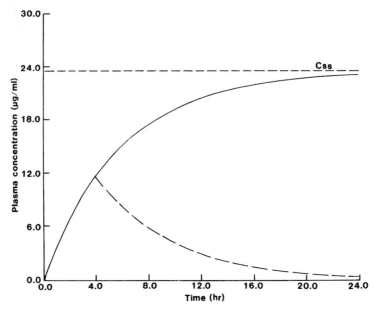

Figure 3.5 Linear plot of plasma concentration vs. time during a continuous i.v. infusion showing plasma concentration approaching C_{ss} (upper dashed line). Also shown is the calculated plasma concentration if the infusion is stopped at 4 h (lower dashed line)

plasma concentration should be achieved. This steady state plasma concentration (C_{ss}) can be calculated from Equation 3.11.

$$C_{ss} = k_o/(k.V)$$
$$= k_o/CL \qquad (3.11)$$

Finally, the drug concentration at any time after the termination of an infusion (the lower dashed line in Figure 3.5) can be calculated by first calculating the concentration, $C\tau$, at the end of the infusion (τ hours), using Equation 3.10, and then by multiplying this concentration by the exponential term for elimination. The full equation is given:

$$C = C_\tau . e^{-k.t}$$

or

$$C = \frac{k_o}{V.k} . [1 - e^{-k.\tau}] . e^{-k.(t - \mu)} \qquad (3.12)$$

Both forms of this equation are quite similar to Equation 3.6.

Single dose oral or extravascular drug administration

The oral route is the most common method of drug administration. Drugs are also frequently given by intramuscular or subcutaneous injection. Topical, buccal, rectal or inhalational administration may also produce systemic concentrations of drug. All these routes can be described mathematically with a common kinetic model. That is the model shown in Figure 3.1, with an absorption step that follows first order kinetics. The kinetic model for oral administration is shown in Figure 3.6.

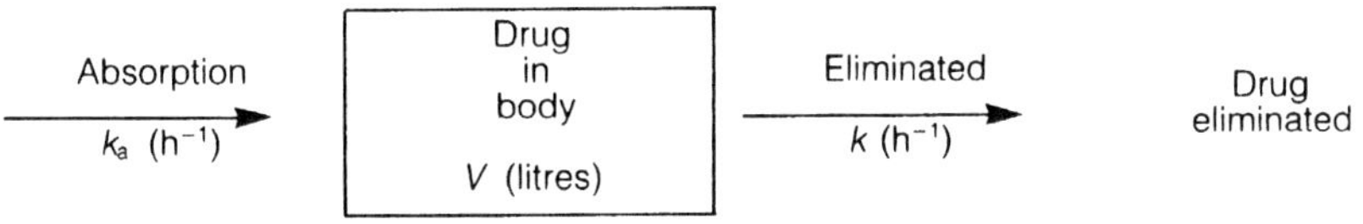

Figure 3.6 Diagram of the one-compartment model showing first order absorption and elimination

The rate of change of C is governed by the rate of absorption and the rate of elimination.

$$dC/dt = \text{Rate in} - \text{Rate out}$$
$$= k_a.A_G/V - k.C \qquad (3.13)$$

where k_a is the first order rate constant for absorption and A_G is the amount of drug remaining to be absorbed from the site of administration at any given time.

Immediately after the dose is administered the plasma concentration is zero and the rate out will be zero. However, the plasma concentration will rise as drug is absorbed, the rate in initially being larger than the rate out. The plasma concentration will eventually peak as the elimination process overtakes the rate of absorption of drug from the site of administration. The rate in is equal to the rate out when the maximum plasma concentration is reached. If no more drug is given the plasma concentration will then progressively fall back to zero, as the rate out now becomes larger than the rate in. The overall plasma concentration vs. time profile can be calculated with Equation 3.14 which is derived from Equation 3.13.

$$C = \frac{F.DOSE.k_a}{V.(k_a-k)}.[e^{-k.t} - e^{-k_a.t}] \qquad (3.14)$$

where F = the fraction of the dose which is absorbed (i.e. the bioavailability).

From Equation 3.14 it is possible to calculate the plasma concentration at any time after the oral, i.m., subcutaneous or any other extravascular drug administration. Typical plasma concentration vs. time curves are shown in Figures 3.7 and 3.8.

Michaelis–Menten kinetics

The capacity of all enzymatic processes is limited and the metabolism of

47

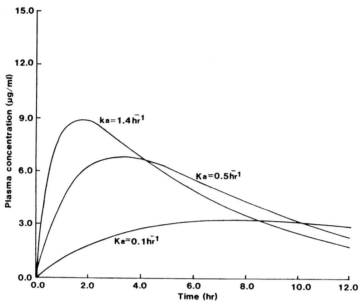

Figure 3.7 Linear plot of plasma concentration vs. time after extravascular drug administration. The effect of varying the absorption rate constant value is shown by the three solid lines

some drugs can become capacity limited at high therapeutic drug plasma concentrations. For these drugs the metabolic elimination step is better represented by Michaelis–Menten kinetics rather than by a first order rate process. The maximum velocity of the process, V_m, and the Michaelis–Menten constant, K_m, can be used in the rate equation to mathematically describe the metabolism step. The equations for the rate of change of plasma concentration after i.v. bolus, i.v. infusion, and oral administration, all with Michaelis–Menten elimination, are given in Equations 3.15, 3.16, and 3.17, respectively.

$$dC/dt = - V_m.C/(K_m + C) \qquad (3.15)$$

$$dC/dt = k_o/V - V_m.C/(K_m + C) \qquad (3.16)$$

$$dC/dt = k_a.A_G/V - V_m.C/(K_m + C) \qquad (3.17)$$

Although Equations 3.15, 3.16 and 3.17 cannot be integrated algebraically, plasma concentration vs. time curves can be calculated from them by computer using numerical integration methods. The two plasma concentration vs. time curves (plotted semilogarithmically) in Figure 3.9 illustrate the effect of Michaelis–Menten kinetics after a single rapid i.v. administration of a drug. The lower curve has been calculated with a dose producing plasma concentrations low enough for apparent first order kinetics to be observed, whereas the top curve clearly indicates non-linear or non-first

48

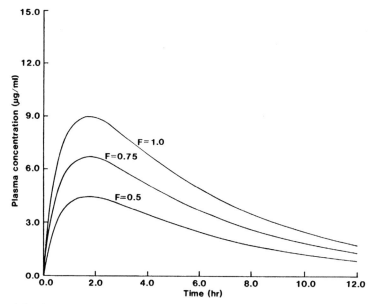

Figure 3.8 Linear plot of plasma concentration vs. time after extravascular drug administration. In this figure the effect of varying the value of F is shown

order elimination kinetics when a higher dose is used. This non-linearity is highlighted by plotting the curves as log C vs. time. First order elimination produces a straight line, whereas the Michaelis–Menten process produces a line which changes progressively from a curved (zero order) part to a straight line (first order) region, as concentration falls. At high concentrations, when C is much larger than K_m, Equation 3.15 approximates that of zero order elimination, with $dC/dt = -V_m$ since K_m+C becomes almost equal to C. At low concentrations, with C much less than K_m, Equation 3.15 becomes virtually a first order equation, $dC/dt = -(V_m/K_m).C$ (since K_m+C becomes almost identical with K_m), with (V_m/K_m) a pseudo first order rate constant.

TWO-COMPARTMENT MODELS

As has already been pointed out the distribution of many drugs between the central vascular compartment and the peripheral tissues is either quite rapid or relatively insignificant in magnitude. In either case the kinetic model of a one-compartment pharmacokinetic model is quite sufficient to describe the plasma concentration vs. time data measured at the usual sampling times possible in studies in man. However, if drug distribution is extensive or relatively slow and if plasma samples are collected at early and at frequent intervals, it is often possible to observe two phases, an early rapid and a subsequent slow phase, in the plasma concentration vs. time curve. In general, it is then sufficient to use a two-compartment model

49

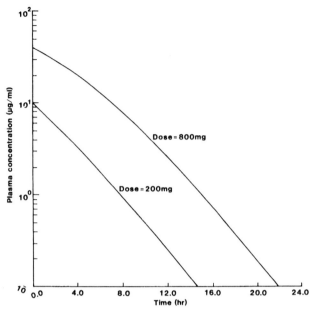

Figure 3.9 Semilogarithmic plot of plasma concentration vs. time after a single i.v. bolus dose for a drug exhibiting Michaelis–Menten elimination kinetics. The upper line shows the increased departure from a straight line as early concentration values are well above the K_m value

in representing the body, but three- or four- compartment models have been used for some drugs when extensive early plasma concentration vs. time observations have been made. For the present we will confine the discussion to a two-compartment pharmacokinetic model, which is represented schematically in Figure 3.10.

Notice that muscle is included in both compartments in Figure 3.10. Inclusion of a particular tissue depends on individual circumstances and for some drugs one tissue may be a fast equilibrating tissue and for other drugs the same tissue may be in a slowly equilibrating compartment. The number of compartments required to describe the observed data is determined empirically and generally no precise anatomical assignment is attempted. In the simplest representation of the two-compartment pharmacokinetic model all the rate constants are first order.

Single rapid i.v. injection

Again we can begin by considering the simplest case, i.e. that of a drug administered by rapid i.v. injection. Assuming that the drug is rapidly mixed in the plasma of the patient the initial plasma concentration can be calculated by dividing the dose by the apparent volume of distribution for the central compartment.

$$C(0) = \text{DOSE}/V_1 \tag{3.18}$$

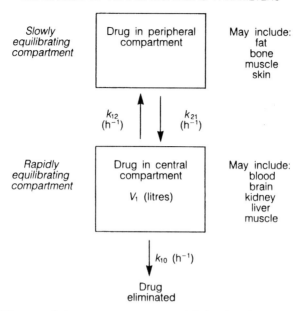

Figure 3.10 Diagram of the two-compartment model showing distribution of drug into peripheral tissues and elimination

Once the drug is in the circulation it may undergo excretion, metabolism and distribution between the central and peripheral compartments. The change in plasma concentration can then be expressed by the rate equation, Equation 3.19, where k_{10} represents all the elimination steps, both excretion and metabolism.

$$dC/dt = -(k_{10} + k_{12}).C + k_{21}.A_T/V_1 \qquad (3.19)$$

where A_T/V_1 represents the amount of drug in the peripheral compartment divided by V_1.

This equation can be integrated to give a biexponential equation, Equation 3.20, for plasma concentration as a function of time.

$$C = A.e^{-\alpha.t} + B.e^{-\beta.t} \qquad (3.20)$$

with $\alpha > \beta$.

The A, B, α, and β terms are functions of k_{10}, k_{12}, k_{21}, V_1, and dose. The two terms, α and β, reflect the slopes of the two phases into which the plasma concentration vs. time curve can be decomposed. A typical two-compartment plasma concentration vs. time curve is shown in Figure 3.11.

Once A, B, α, and β are calculated from the plasma concentration vs. time curve (see Chapter 4), the rate constants k_{10}, k_{21}, and k_{12} can be readily calculated.

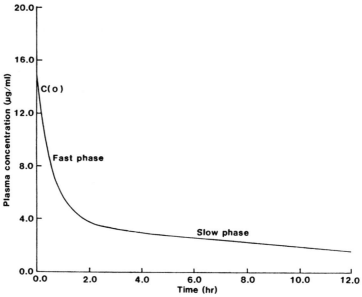

Figure 3.11 Linear plot of plasma concentration vs. time calculated according to the two-compartment model. The biexponential nature of this curve is shown as fast and slow phases

$$k_{10} = \frac{\alpha.\beta. \ (A + B)}{A.\beta + B.\alpha} \tag{3.21}$$

$$k_{12} = \frac{A.B.(\beta - \alpha)^2}{(A + B).(A.\beta + B.\alpha)} \tag{3.22}$$

$$k_{21} = \frac{A.\beta + B.\alpha}{A + B} \tag{3.23}$$

With the one-compartment pharmacokinetic model only one apparent volume of distribution could be calculated. However, for the two-compartment model, a number of different apparent volumes can be determined.

$$V_1 = DOSE/ \ (A + B) \tag{3.24}$$

$$V_\beta = DOSE/ \ (\beta.AUC)$$

$$= V_1.k_{10}/\beta$$
$$= CL/\beta \tag{3.25}$$

$$V_{extrap} = DOSE/B \tag{3.26}$$

$$V_{ss} = V_1.(k_{12}+k_{21})/k_{21} \tag{3.27}$$

where AUC is the calculated area under the complete plasma concentration vs. time curve. This term can be calculated using the trapezoidal rule as described in Chapter 4.

The volume of the central compartment, V_1, determines the value of $C(0)$ after a rapid i.v. dose. Therefore the maximum expected plasma concentration can be determined. The value of V_β, also known as V_{area} is easily determined and can be useful for calculating dosing regimens. The V_{extrap} value is determined if the distribution phase is ignored. Finally, V steady state, V_{ss}, gives a measure of the apparent volume of the central plus the peripheral compartment. It can be used to determine the total amount of drug in the body once a pseudo equilibrium is established between the peripheral and central compartments.

Single i.v. infusion

For various reasons (see above) it may be desirable to give a drug by intravenous infusion. If the infusion process is added to the rate Equation 3.19 and then integrated, it is possible to obtain an equation for the plasma concentration vs. time curve during and after a single i.v. infusion with a two-compartment model. This equation is given below (Equation 3.28).

$$C \;=\; \frac{k_o.(k_{21} - \alpha).(1 - e^{\alpha.\tau}).e^{-\alpha.t}}{V_1.\alpha.(\alpha - \beta)}$$
$$+\; \frac{k_o.(\beta - k_{21}).(1 - e^{\beta.\tau}).e^{-\beta.t}}{V_1.\beta.(\alpha - \beta)} \tag{3.28}$$

During the infusion period, τ is equal to time, t, and thus varies with time. However, once the infusion is terminated the value of τ becomes fixed as the duration of the infusion. A typical plasma curve achieved after an extended i.v. infusion with a two-compartment distribution model is shown in Figure 3.12.

This figure illustrates the increase in plasma concentration with a continuous infusion. Because drug distribution is an important part of drug disposition, when a two-compartment model is involved, the time to reach a steady state concentration can be quite long. The steady state concentration after a prolonged infusion can be determined from Equation 3.28. The equation is the same as 3.11.

$$\begin{aligned} C_{ss} &= k_o/(k_{10}.V_1) \\ &= k_o/(V_\beta.\beta) \end{aligned} \tag{3.29}$$

If the infusion is terminated after a relatively short infusion period, such as 1 or 2 h, a fast phase will be seen to precede the slow phase in the declining plasma concentration vs. time curve. This is shown in the semilog plot of Figure 3.13.

After an infusion of a longer duration the peripheral compartments tend

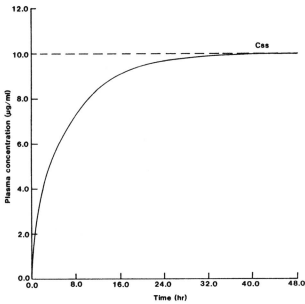

Figure 3.12   Linear plot of plasma concentration vs. time during a continuous i.v. infusion, calculated according to the two-compartment model

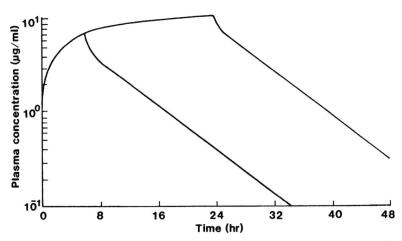

Figure 3.13 Semilogarithmic plot of plasma concentration vs. time after an i.v. infusion stopped at 6 h and 24 h. The biphasic nature of the postinfusion period is less marked after the longer infusion

to be 'filled up' and a pseudo equilibrium is achieved between the drug in the central and peripheral compartments. If the infusion is then terminated a single exponential curve, depicting a combination of redistribution and elimination, would be observed. This is shown in Figure 3.13, calculated after cessation of a 24 h infusion.

One serious difficulty with infusion therapy is the time it takes to achieve a desired steady state plasma concentration. One way to alleviate this problem is to give a short i.v. infusion or bolus dose before the main slower sustaining infusion. If a rapid injection is used before the infusion the combined effect can be calculated by combining Equations 3.20 and 3.28.

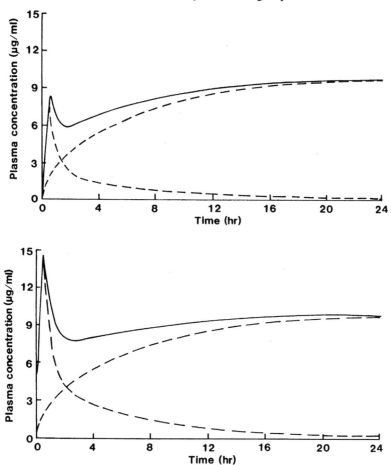

Figure 3.14 Linear plot of plasma concentration vs. time after a rapid and slow i.v. infusion of drug given to achieve a rapid approach to C_{ss}. (a) An approach from below C_{ss}; (b) the result of a faster initial infusion with approach from above C_{ss}

A typical combined curve is shown in Figure 3.14 along with the composite curves for a single rapid injection and a single sustaining infusion. In Figure 3.14 two different values are used for the single rapid infusion dose. In each case the plasma concentration approached the steady state value more quickly than with a single infusion, the lower dashed line. In one case

(Figure 3.14b) the more rapid approach is from above the steady state level, in the other (Figure 3.14a) the approach is slower but lower plasma concentrations are present. The disadvantage of the approach from above is that it may involve potentially toxic plasma concentrations.

If a drug follows two-compartmental pharmacokinetics it is not possible to match the steady state plasma concentration with a single i.v. bolus dose. In some cases it may be possible to use a series of small rapid injections or infusions to achieve a therapeutic concentration of drug rapidly. This is often done empirically by the physician when a drug has a clearly measurable pharmacological action, as is the case with the muscle relaxants. If the empirical approach is used it is important to remember that the incremental doses are at least in part intended to replace drug which has distributed out of the central compartment rather than been eliminated from the body. Prolonged pharmacological effect or toxic overdosage may be the outcome of repeated empirical dosing.

Single dose oral or other extramuscular administration

For a drug which appears to follow a one-compartment pharmacokinetic model, the plasma concentration vs. time curve after oral administration can be described by a biexponential equation, Equation 3.14. For a drug following two-compartment pharmacokinetics after extravascular administration, the corresponding equation is triexponential. The α, β and the absorption rate constants all contribute exponential terms to the overall equation. The equation for plasma concentration as a function of time is given by Equation 3.30.

$$C = A.e^{-\alpha.t} + B.e^{-\beta.t} - (A+B).e^{-k_a.t} \qquad (3.30)$$

As before α and β are hybrid constants with $\alpha > \beta$.

According to this equation it should be possible to recognize a triexponential curve for plasma concentration as a function of time after oral administration. Whether this is possible in practice depends on the values of the three parameters α, β, and k_a. If these parameters are sufficiently different, three exponentials may be evident in the plasma concentration vs. time curve. This is shown in the semilog plot of Figure 3.15. Also shown in Figure 3.15 is a curve calculated with the α and k_a values fairly close. The first line exhibits three exponentials, while in the second line only two exponentials are apparent. In later chapters we will discuss methods of separating the three exponentials, even when two of them have similar values so that their effect cannot readily be distinguished by eye.

Michaelis–Menten elimination kinetics

For some drugs it may be necessary to include Michaelis–Menten kinetics in the pharmacokinetic model in addition to a peripheral distribution compartment. Again algebraic integration of differential equations is not possible. However, the plasma concentration vs. time profiles can be calculated by numerical integration of the differential equations.

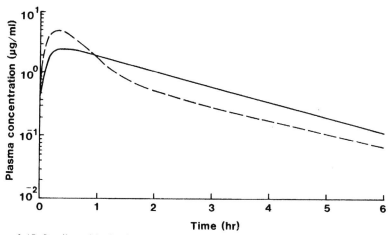

Figure 3.15 Semilogarithmic plot of plasma concentration vs. time after extravascular drug administration, calculated according to the two-compartment model. The dashed line illustrates a curve calculated with quite different values of α, β, and k_a whereas the solid line was calculated with α and k_a closer in value

MULTIPLE DRUG ADMINISTRATIONS

When a drug is given for testing purposes or for acute treatment a single dose may be appropriate. However, most drugs are given in multiple dose regimens. That is, repeated doses of a drug are given to achieve therapeutic activity, e.g. to continuously combat the symptoms of a disease, to completely eradicate an infecting organism, or to maintain a steady prophylactic plasma and tissue drug concentration for long-term management of a disease state. Repeated drug administration leads to accumulation of the drug in the patient's body. With properly spaced drug administration the accumulation of drug can be controlled to produce the desired plasma concentration vs. time profile.

Multiple intravenous administrations

When drug doses are spaced widely enough, all the drug from the first dose may be completely eliminated before the second dose is given. Accumulation will not occur; it will be as though two separate single doses were given. The plasma concentration during each dosing interval may be calculated using the single dose equations discussed earlier. The plasma curve after repeated widely spaced i.v. injections (every 24 h) of a drug with a 4 h halflife is shown in Figure 3.16.

This situation can be contrasted with the plasma concentration curve after more closely spaced intravenous drug administrations. If the drug in the previous example had been given once every elimination halflife, i.e. every 4 h, the second and subsequent doses would have been given while half of the drug from the previous doses was still in the body. Immediately after the second i.v. dose, the plasma concentration would be 150% of that

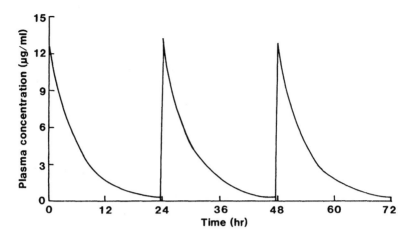

Figure 3.16 Linear plot of plasma concentration vs. time after multiple i.v. bolus doses, calculated according to the one-compartment model. No accumulation is shown as the dose times are well separated

immediately after the first dose. Immediately after the third dose, the plasma concentration would be 175% higher than after the first dose, after the fourth dose 187.5%, and so on. This situation is illustrated by the concentration vs. time curve in Figure 3.17.

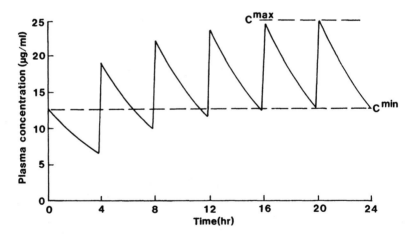

Figure 3.17 Linear plot of plasma concentration vs. time after more frequent multiple i.v. doses. Plasma concentrations are shown to accumulate, approaching C^{max} and C^{min} values at the start and the end of each dosing interval

The equation for this type of curve can be easily derived for multiple intravenous doses. At the end of the first dosing interval the plasma concentration is given by Equation 3.31.

$$C = (DOSE/V).exp^{(-k.\tau)} \tag{3.31}$$

$$= (DOSE/V).(0.5) \text{ in the example above}$$

where τ is the dosing interval. If the dosing interval is equal to the elimination halflife (4 h in this example) the term $e^{-k.\tau}$ is equal to 0.5. When the dosing interval is not equal to the elimination halflife it is convenient to substitute R for the term $e^{-k.\tau}$ to simplify the algebra. Now the plasma concentration at the end of the first interval is given by Equation 3.32.

$$C_{\tau,1} = (DOSE/V).R \tag{3.32}$$

Note that in Equation 3.32 and subsequent equations the first subscript (τ) refers to the time since the last dose and the second subscript (1) refers to the dose number.

Immediately after the second intravenous dose the plasma concentration is:

$$C_{0,2} = (DOSE/V).R + (DOSE/V) \tag{3.33}$$

and at the end of the second dosing interval

$$C_{\tau,2} = (DOSE/V).R^2 + (DOSE/V).R \tag{3.34}$$

This sequence of equations can be repeated for any number of equal doses given at equal dosing intervals, τ. The plasma concentration at the beginning and end of the 'n'th dosing interval can be calculated as follows.

$$C_{0,n} = (DOSE/V).R^{(n-1)} + (DOSE/V).R^{(n-2)} + \ldots$$
$$+ (DOSE/V) \tag{3.35}$$

and

$$C_{\tau,n} = (DOSE/V).R^n + (DOSE/V).R^{(n-1)} + \ldots$$
$$(DOSE/V).R \tag{3.36}$$

Equations 3.35 and 3.36 can be simplified by recognizing that they represent the sum of two geometric series. Therefore these equations can be replaced by Equations 3.37 and 3.38.

$$C_{0,n} = (DOSE/V).\frac{[1 - R^n]}{[1 - R]} \tag{3.37}$$

and

$$C_{\tau,n} \quad = \quad (\text{DOSE}/V) . \frac{[1-R^n]}{[1 - R]} .R \qquad (3.38)$$

Since the plasma concentration at any time, t, during the dosing interval is equal to the plasma concentration at the start of the interval multiplied by $e^{-k.t}$, Equation 3.39 can be derived.

$$C_{t,n} \quad = \quad (\text{DOSE}/V) . \frac{[1 - R^n]}{[1 - R]} .\exp^{-k.t} \qquad (3.39)$$

This equation can be used to calculate the plasma concentration at any time, t, after any number of doses, n, given by rapid intravenous injection. A typical plasma concentration vs. time curve during a 12 h multiple dose regimen is shown in Figure 3.18.

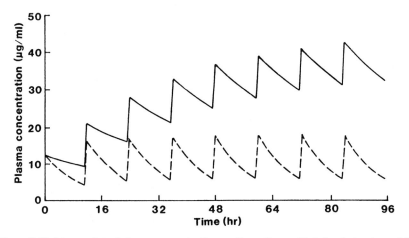

Figure 3.18 Linear plot of plasma concentration vs. time after multiple i.v. bolus doses. The dashed line shows the effect of a larger k value on drug accumulation

This figure illustrates the accumulation of drug in the body after a number of doses. Repeated drug administration, with a fixed dose per dosing interval, is analogous to the continuous i.v. infusion with an approach to a steady state plasma concentration. In the case of multiple dose administration the plasma concentration fluctuates between a minimum and maximum concentration during each dosing interval. These minimum and maximum values are described by Equations 3.40 and 3.41, for repeated i.v. bolus doses. Like the continuous infusion, the plasma concentration rises to a plateau level, though with the concentration fluctuating between a maximum, C_{max}, and a minimum, C_{min}, value after a sufficient time (the time to achieve a steady state).

$$C_{max} = \frac{\text{DOSE}}{V.(1-R)} \qquad (3.40)$$

$$C_{min} = \frac{\text{DOSE}.R}{V.(1-R)} \qquad (3.41)$$

Multiple oral drug administrations

Multiple drug administration most commonly occurs by the oral route. The inclusion of a first order absorption step further complicates the equation for plasma concentration as a function of time. In this situation the most useful equation is one used to calculate the average plasma concentration achieved at steady state (C_{av}) during a multiple drug regimen which has been continued long enough for steady state conditions to apply. This equation is valid if linear pharmacokinetics apply and if k does not change with time.

$$C_{av} = \frac{F.\text{DOSE}}{V.k.\tau} = \frac{F.\text{DOSE}}{CL.\tau} \qquad (3.42)$$

With this equation it is possible to calculate a suitable maintenance dose to achieve any desired average steady state plasma concentration. It is worth noting that the same average plasma concentration is achieved if the dose and dosing interval, τ, are altered in the same proportion. For example, if the dose is changed from 300 mg every 6 h to 600 mg every 12 h, the same average plasma concentration will result, again assuming that linear kinetics apply. However, the maximum and minimum concentrations would be more widely varied with the longer dosing interval. This effect is illustrated in Figure 3.19.

When uniform doses are given at uniform dosing intervals Equation 3.42 can be used to calculate either a dose and dosing interval needed, or the expected average plasma concentration from a uniform dosing regimen.

Unfortunately, dosing regimens are not always uniform in practice, especially when oral drug administration is involved. A typical dosage regimen of one tablet three times a day may mean that the patient takes the medication at 8 a.m., 12 noon, and 6 p.m. With such a schedule the dosing intervals are 4, 6, and 14 h throughout the 24 h period. This can mean a reduced plasma drug concentration overnight and in the early morning as illustrated in Figure 3.20.

For the treatment of some symptoms such a regimen may be sufficient. However, for other situations (e.g. antibiotic therapy) more even maintenance of therapeutic plasma concentrations may be essential. The dosing regimen must then be organized with more care. If the patient was instructed to take the medication at 7 a.m., 3 p.m. and 11 p.m. an 8 h dosing interval could be maintained. The effect of this alternative dosing regimen is also shown in Figure 3.20.

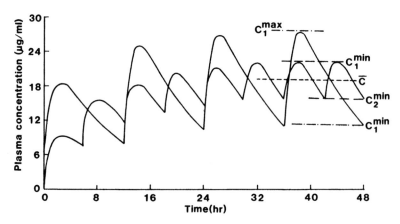

Figure 3.19 Linear plot of plasma concentration vs. time after multiple extravascular doses. Illustrated is the wider range between $C_{1\,max}$ and $C_{1\,min}$ after 12 hourly dosing compared with the narrower range after 6 hourly dosing. Note that $\bar{C}$ is the same in each case

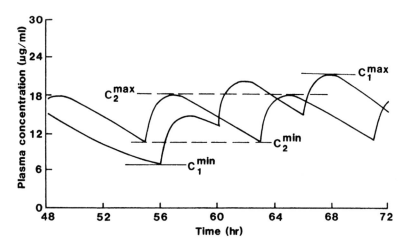

Figure 3.20 Linear plot of plasma concentration vs. time after multiple extravascular doses. The wider range between $C_{1\,max}$ and $C_{1\,min}$ results from the non-uniform dosing intervals. The plasma concentration variations are reduced when a uniform dosing interval is used

4
Determination of pharmacokinetic parameters from laboratory data

In the previous chapter many equations were presented which describe the plasma concentration vs. time profiles that result from various patterns of drug administration. Armed with values for the relevant parameters and with a knowledge of the appropriate pharmacokinetic model the calculation of plasma concentration vs. time profiles is straightforward, if somewhat tedious. In this chapter we will tackle the reverse problem, that of determining values for some of the various pharmacokinetic parameters already described, when plasma concentration vs. time data are available after an experimental study.

It is sometimes possible to obtain quite good estimates of pharmacokinetic parameters with little more than a piece of graph paper and a ruler. In other cases more sophisticated methods such as non-linear regression analysis are necessary. In this chapter various approaches will be discussed, with some indication of the limitations of each method considered.

ONE-COMPARTMENT PHARMACOKINETIC MODEL

I.V. bolus

Plasma concentration vs. time data collected after a rapid intravenous dose of a drug should be the easiest to analyse. If it is already known that a drug follows one-compartment linear kinetics it is possible to determine both k and V after the collection of as few as two accurate plasma concentration vs. time values. (It would be impossible to know whether a one-compartment model was valid if only two sets of plasma concentration vs. time data were available.) The two observations can be plotted on semilog graph paper, according to Equation 4.1, and a straight line drawn through the points. Equation 4.1 was derived from Equation 3.5 by taking logarithms (base 10) of both sides of Equation 3.5.

$$\log(C) = \log(C(0)) - k.t/2.3 \qquad (4.1)$$

Extrapolation of the line to zero time on the concentration axis gives the value for $C(0)$. The apparent volume of distribution can be calculated as $V = DOSE/C(0)$. The slope of the line can be calculated from the two determinations as slope $= [\log(C_1) - \log(C_2)]/(t_1 - t_2)$. If in this calculation of the slope, logarithms to the base 10 are used the elimination rate constant can be calculated from the slope of the line as $k = -2.3 \times$slope (as $2.3 = \ln(10)$, base e). In these days of hand-held calculators and personal microcomputers, it is easier to calculate k directly as $k = -[\ln(C_1) - \ln(C_2)]/(t_1 - t_2)$ when logarithms to the base e are used. An alternative calculation of k can be made via the value of the elimination halflife. By definition the elimination halflife of a first order process is the time taken for the concentration to fall to one half of its original value. This time value can be read from the graph (for instance, as the time to reach half the $C(0)$ value). The elimination halflife can now be calculated as $k = 0.693/t_\frac{1}{2} = \ln(2)/t_\frac{1}{2}$ (Equation 3.7).

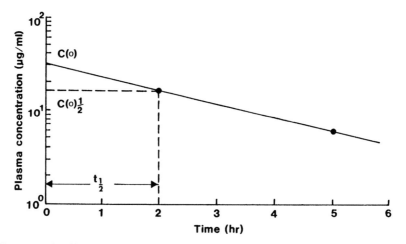

Figure 4.1 Semilogarithmic plot of plasma concentration vs. time illustrating the determination of $C(0)$ and $t_\frac{1}{2}$

These calculations are illustrated in the semilog plot of Figure 4.1 and in the example calculation.

Two plasma concentration determinations were made at 2 and 5 h after a rapid intravenous injection of 250 mg drug. These values, 15.4 and 5.7 μg/ml, respectively, are shown in Figure 4.1. The two points are connected by a line drawn back to the concentration axis. From this line the $C(0)$ value can be determined as 30 μg/ml. Consequently the apparent volume of distribution can be calculated as DOSE/C(0) or 250/30 = 8.33 l.

The elimination rate constant can be calculated directly as $-[\ln(15.4)-\ln(5.7)]/(2-5) = 0.331$ h^{-1}. Alternatively, the elimination halflife can be estimated from the graph as 2.05 h and the elimination rate constant calculated as 0.338 h^{-1}.

Determination of 'best fit' line by 'eye'

Accurate determinations of k and V using only two data points are possible only if the data are very accurate, and a simple one-compartment model is known to apply. A more general approach is to use multiple data points collected at carefully selected times. For a drug following a one-compartment pharmacokinetic model, four to six accurate data points collected after a rapid intravenous injection should allow the determination of accurate parameter values and confirmation of the model. Again, the data points should fall on or close to a straight line when plotted on semilog graph paper. Rarely, in practice, will all the data fall exactly on a straight line. However, a line of 'best fit' can be drawn through the data, judging by 'eye' the position of the line. This 'best fit' line can be extended to the y-axis as above, $C(0)$ measured and V can again be calculated as DOSE/$C(0)$. The elimination rate constant can also be calculated from this line by using two points on the line as drawn, towards each end, to calculate the slope.

$$\text{Slope} = \frac{[\log(C_{\text{at one end}}) - \log(C_{\text{at other end}}]}{[t_{\text{at one end}} - t_{\text{at other end}}]}$$

The elimination rate constant, k, can then be calculated as $-2.3 \times$ slope. Choosing a line of 'best fit' by eye can often give quite good answers. However, it is a subjective method, and different people may calculate quite different answers from the one set of data. Also, when the data are plotted on semilog graph paper the tendency is to give the lower concentrations more emphasis than may be warranted. The accuracy of lower concentration determinations may be somewhat less than that of the higher concentration values. It is hard to be completely objective when determining the 'best fit' line by eye.

Semilog linear regression

Rather than simply determining the line by 'eye', semilog linear regression analysis can be used to calculate the slope and intercept of the 'best fit' line. This method will provide not only values for the parameters V and k but also will give estimates of (1) how well the line describes the data, and (2) the uncertainty in the parameter values determined. The usually applied linear regression methods assume that the time values are accurately known and that the probable error in each experimentally determined concentration value is the same. Therefore the regression method usually gives each data point the same weight or emphasis.

This regression method can be illustrated by analysing the set of data in Table 4.1.

Table 4.1

Time (h)	Plasma concentration (μg/ml)	ln(C)
1	22.3	3.105
2	17.0	2.833
4	14.0	2.639
6	10.3	2.332
9	6.9	1.932
12	3.4	1.224

This data set was generated by calculating accurate plasma concentrations using Equation 3.6 with $k = 0.17$ h^{-1}; $V = 4$ l; and dose = 100 mg. To each calculated point was added a normally distributed random error multiplied by 10% of each accurate value. This means that the uncertainty in each value is proportional to the value itself. This is the usual situation when the concentration determined is well within the assay sensitivity limits. That is, the error is random but proportional to the concentration value.

If we first take the logarithm of each concentration value (Table 4.1, column 3) we can now calculate a best fit to the $ln(C)$ vs. time data using ordinary linear regression analysis. This analysis assumes that there is no error in the time value determinations (the 'x' term) and is usually performed with the assumption that the error in the y term (in this case $ln(C)$) is the same for all y values. This means that the error in C is assumed to be proportional to the C value (because of the logarithmic transformation). As this was how the error was added to the data we should expect to calculate fairly accurate values for k and V. By normal linear regression of $ln(C)$ vs. time, the slope (or k) value proved to be 0.16 h^{-1} and the intercept value was 3.25 (= 25.84 μg/ml); thus $V = 3.87$ l.

Non-linear regression analysis

Another method of data analysis is non-linear regression analysis. With this method the parameters of Equation 3.6 are adjusted to fit the untransformed equation to the data. The data can be given equal weights (that is, the magnitude of the error in each value is assumed constant) or a weight proportional to the concentration value squared (that is, the standard deviation of the error is proportional to the data), or any number of other weighting schemes depending on the assumed or known error structure for the data. Because of the complexity of the calculation, non-linear regression analysis is usually performed with the aid of a relatively large computer program, such as the so-called NONLIN, NLIN or SAAM, although microcomputer programs such as MULTI (*see* Appendix) are now available for this purpose. These computer programs determine a 'weighted best fit' to the data by iteratively altering the parameter values until the weighted sum of squares (WSS) is minimized. The WSS value is calculated by multiplying the weight given to each point by the square of the difference between the calculated concentration and the experimental concentration. That is:

$$\text{WSS} = \Sigma_{i=1}^{i=n} [\text{weight}_i * (\text{Calcd}_i - \text{Experimental}_i)^2]$$

The information required to perform a non-linear fit includes the data, a weighting scheme and initial estimates for all of the parameters of the model to be fitted to the data. In the case of the i.v. bolus data given in Table 4.1 a weighting scheme of (1) equal weight and (2) weight proportional to the square of each concentration value were used in two separate calculations. The 'best fit' parameter values obtained by the semilog regression above were used as initial estimates. The plasma data were fitted to the model shown in Scheme 4.1. The lines of BASIC computer code shown in Scheme 4.1 are included in the MULTI non-linear fitting program described in the Appendix.

```
1010 CP = CN(1)* EXP (−P(1)*T) / P(2): RETURN
1011 REM P(1) = KEL:P(2) = V:CN(1) = DOSE
11610 M = 2:NC = 1:PL$(1) = "KEL":PL$(2) = "V":CN$(1) =
         "DOSE":MD$ = "ONE COMPARTMENT-I.V. BOLUS": GOTO
         11700
```

Scheme 4.1

Using the equal weight scheme the values of k and V were 0.152 h^{-1} and 4.00 l, whereas with the other weighting scheme the 'best fit' values were 0.161 h^{-1} and 3.88 l. The coefficients of multiple determination values, r^2, for each fit were 0.985 and 1.000, respectively. In this relatively simple case we can see the effect of different weighting schemes. Both schemes appear to yield satisfactory results considering the 10% error in the data. The r^2 value is a measure of how well the fitted line explains the data and can be interpreted as a fraction of an ideal fit. Therefore, it appears that the fit generated by the two weighting schemes can explain 98.5 or 100% of the data, respectively. The effect of the weighting scheme is also shown in Figure 4.2 which presents the data and the two regression lines calculated using the two different weighting schemes.

As can be seen, for this set of data either line validly describes the experimental data. With more complicated pharmacokinetic models the selection of an appropriate weighting scheme becomes more important. In the case of non-linear fitting selection of the model, the weighting scheme, and estimation of initial parameter values, are important steps to a satisfactory fit to the experimental data.

Area under the plasma concentration vs. time curve (AUC)

The area under the plasma concentration vs. time curve (AUC) is an

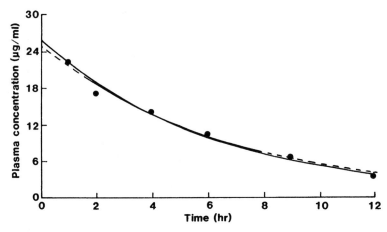

Figure 4.2 Linear plot of plasma concentration vs. time showing best fit lines and data points. The solid line was calculated with the equal weight scheme and the dashed line was calculated with the other weighting scheme

important parameter used in the determination of the relative bioavailability of dosage forms and other parameter calculations. The AUC after i.v. bolus administration is often used as a reference value for oral or other extravascular dosage forms. The usual method of calculating the AUC value is by trapezoidal rule integration. By this procedure the total area under the plasma concentration vs. time curve is broken up into smaller consecutive trapezoidal segments. If we take the data presented in Table

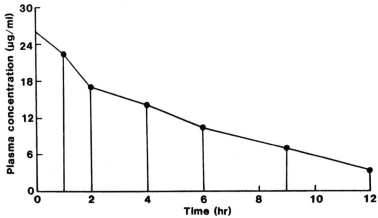

Figure 4.3 Linear plot of plasma concentration vs. time illustrating the trapezoids used to make up the area under the curve

4.1 as an example, plotted again in Figure 4.3, we can break the total area into seven segments. Five of these segments, defined by the six data points, have shapes approximated by trapezoids. The area of each trapezoid shape can then be calculated as the base $(t_{i+1} - t_i)$ multiplied by the average height $(C_i + C_{i+1})/2$. For the first segment the area would be:

$$\begin{aligned}
\text{Area} &= (2 - 1) \times (22.3 + 17.0)/2 \\
&= 1 \times 39.3/2 \\
&= 19.65\,\mu\text{g h ml}^{-1}
\end{aligned}$$

In a similar fashion the area of each of the five segments can be calculated and the sum of the individual values obtained. Alternative methods have to be employed for the first and last segment. For the first segment an extrapolated value of $C(0)$ is necessary and can be calculated by semilog regression analysis or by the method of drawing a 'best fit' line by eye. Either method would give a value close to 26 μg/ml for $C(0)$. The area of this first trapezoid can now be calculated as for the other five segments. This value is shown in Table 4.2.

Table 4.2

Time (h)	Plasma concentration (μg/ml)	AUC (μg hml^{-1})
0	(26.0)	–
1	22.3	24.15
2	17.0	19.65
4	14.0	31.00
6	10.3	24.30
9	6.9	25.80
12	3.4	15.45
infinity	0.0	21.25
		Total AUC 161.99

The final segment, from the last data point to infinite time, can be calculated if we assume that the plasma concentration will continue to decline monoexponentially from the last data point. Integrating the equation for monoexponential decline yields the same result as calculating the area under the curve. Thus:

$$C = C_{\text{last}}.e^{-k'.t}$$

where k' is the rate constant for the monoexponential decline. For this case $k' = k$. Integrating both sides gives:

$$\text{Area of last segment} = C_{\text{last}}/k$$

Using the value for k determined by the semilog regression analysis (0.16 h^{-1}) and the last measured C value (3.4 μg/ml) the area of the last segment can be calculated as 3.4/0.16 or 21.25 μg h ml^{-1}. The total area under the plasma concentration vs. time curve is now calculated by summing the areas of the individual segments, as in Table 4.2.

In the case of an i.v. bolus administration the total AUC value can be more easily calculated by taking advantage of the monoexponential decay in the plasma concentration vs. time curve. Just as the AUC of the last segment can be calculated as C_{last}/k, the total AUC can be calculated as $C(0)/k$. Thus the total AUC could be calculated as 26/0.16 or 162.5 μg h ml^{-1}.

Total body clearance

Once the AUC value is determined it is possible to calculate the total body clearance (CL) and in fact this calculation is valid irrespective of the particular pharmacokinetic model which applies so long as linear kinetics apply. After i.v. bolus drug administration the CL can be determined as DOSE/AUC. For the above example this is:

$$\begin{aligned} CL &= DOSE/AUC \\ &= 100/161 \\ &= 0.621 \text{ l/h} \\ &= 10.4 \text{ ml/min} \end{aligned}$$

An alternative method of calculating CL uses the parameter values for k and V. From Equation 3.8 CL is equal to $k.V$, thus:

$$\begin{aligned} CL &= k.V \\ &= 0.16 \times 3.87 \\ &= 0.619 \text{ l/h} \\ &= 10.3 \text{ ml/min} \end{aligned}$$

This latter method applies only to a one-compartment model whereas the previous method is generally applicable, irrespective of the number of compartments in the pharmacokinetic model.

I.V. infusion

Because there is no absorption step in this model and the infusion rate should be known, the determination of pharmacokinetic parameters after an i.v. infusion is relatively straightforward. Once the infusion has stopped the plasma concentration will fall monoexponentially if a linear one-compartment model is applicable. If two or more plasma concentration determinations were made after the infusion was finished a line of 'best fit' could be drawn through the data plotted on semilog graph paper. This could be drawn by 'eye' or calculated by semilog linear regression as described above. The elimination rate constant could then be calculated from the slope of the line as before. Because the drug is eliminated from the time the infusion is started the back extrapolated intercept value is no longer equal to DOSE/V. From Equation 3.12 the following relationships can be derived:

$$C = \frac{k_o}{V.k} \cdot [1 - e^{-k.\tau}] \cdot e^{-k.(t-\tau)}$$

at t = 0

$$C_{intercept} = \frac{k_o}{V.k} \cdot [1 - e^{-k.\tau}] \cdot e^{-k.\tau}$$

or

$$V = \frac{k_o \cdot [e^{k.\tau - 1}]}{k.C_{intercept}} \qquad (4.2)$$

Since k_o and τ for the infusion are known, once a value for k has been determined it is possible to calculate V, the apparent volume of distribution.

Table 4.3

Time (h)	Plasma concentration (μg/ml)	ln(C)
0	0.0	–
0.25	13.8	2.625
0.5	23.9	3.174
1.0	23.0	3.135
2.0	18.7	2.929
3.0	14.3	2.660
4.0	12.8	2.549
6.0	6.87	1.927
9.0	4.68	1.543
12.0	2.46	0.900

This approach can be examined using the data in Table 4.3 as an example. These data were calculated for an i.v. infusion of 250 mg over 30 min using a value of 0.2 h^{-1} and 10.5 l for k and V, respectively. Again, to each exact data value a random error (mean = 0; SD = 10% of the exact value) was added to give the value in Table 4.3.

If the data in Table 4.3 are plotted on semilog graph paper as in Figure 4.2 a straight line can be drawn through the postinfusion data. By 'eye' a line may be drawn backwards through the y-axis at 28.4 μg/ml with a slope equivalent to $k = 0.211$ h^{-1}. Substituting these values in Equation 4.2 gives a value of 9.28 l for the apparent volume of distribution.

An alternative method of data analysis involves a semilog regression analysis of the postinfusion plasma concentration vs. time data. This analysis using the data in column 3 of Table 4.3 gives an elimination rate constant of 0.201 h^{-1}, and an intercept value of 27.0 μg/ml (corresponding to a volume of distribution value of 9.74 l).

A third method of analysing the data involves a non-linear iterative fitting program such as MULTI. Using the values obtained by 'eye' as initial estimates and a weighting scheme with weight proportional to the data squared, all the data in Table 4.3 were fitted by the equations in Scheme 4.2. The programs lines in Scheme 4.2 are included in the MULTI program described in the Appendix.

1020 TINF = CN(1): IF T<TINF THEN TINF = T
1021 CP = CN(2)∗(1−EXP (−P(1)∗TINF))∗ EXP (−P(1)∗(T−TINF)) / (P(1)∗P(2)): RETURN
1022 REM P(1) = KEL:P(2) = V:CN(1) = INFUSION DURATION:CN(2) = INFUSION RATE
11620 M = 2:NC = 2:PL$(1) = "KEL":PL$(2) = "V":CN$(1) = "T−INF":CN$(2) = "K0":MD$ = "ONE COMPARTMENT-I.V. INFUSION": GOTO 11700

Scheme 4.2

The 'best fit' parameter values were 0.204 h^{-1} and 9.59 l, for k and V, respectively. Using the same initial estimates and equal weights for each data the parameter values were 0.208 h^{-1} and 9.51 l, respectively. The r^2 values were 0.99 and 1.00, respectively. In this example the more appropriate weighting scheme gave slightly better final estimates of the parameter values but the differences were hardly significant, with the method of semilog regression actually giving the most accurate answers.

Oral administration

In this section we include not only oral administration but other extravascular routes of administration, such as intramuscular, subcutaneous, or topical. With this pharmacokinetic situation (which we shall speak of as oral administration, for simplicity) there are four basic parameters to determine. These are k and V as before, but also the absorption rate constant k_a and the extent of absorption (or bioavailability) F. Data analysis involving oral administration can be subdivided into methods for determining the rate of absorption (k_a) and methods for determining the extent of absorption or bioavailability (F), in addition to the previously considered methods of determining the disposition parameters, k and V. As an example of the techniques required to analyse data obtained after oral administration we will consider the concentration vs. time data in Table 4.4. These results were calculated with DOSE = 500 mg, k = 0.25 h^{-1}, k_a = 1.5 h^{-1}, V = 15 l, and F = 0.8.

Again the exact plasma concentration data were calculated and a random error with a standard deviation equal to 10% of the exact value added to produce 'real' data.

Rate constant for absorption, k_a

Method of residuals ('feathering the curve') – In many cases the rate constant for absorption is considerably larger than the rate constant for

Table 4.4

Time (h)	Plasma concentration (μg/ml)
0	0.0
0.25	9.6
0.5	13.8
1.0	19.9
1.5	17.7
2.0	19.8
3.0	15.4
4.0	13.4
6.0	6.5
9.0	3.8
12.0	1.7

elimination. If so, absorption, being the faster process, is complete well before elimination is finished. The practical consequence of this is that at late times (some time after the peak plasma concentration) the plasma concentration vs. time curve decline can be described by the elimination rate constant alone. This can be seen from Equation 3.14. If we rewrite this equation as:

$$C = A'.[e^{-k.t} - e^{-k_a.t}] \qquad (4.3)$$

where

$$A' = \frac{F.DOSE.k_a}{V.(k_a - k)}$$

When k_a is much larger than k the term $\exp(-k_a.t)$ in Equation 4.3 approaches zero much faster than the term $\exp(-k.t)$. At later times the term $\exp(-k_a.t)$ becomes effectively zero. Therefore the Equation 4.4 applies.

$$C_{late} = A'.e^{-k.t} \qquad (4.4)$$

This equation is monoexponential, and is similar to the equation for plasma concentration after an i.v. injection. If the plasma concentration vs. time data are plotted on semilog graph paper, as in Figure 4.4, the late data points will be seen to fall on a straight line (approximately, since the data are not perfect). It is possible to draw a straight line through these late data by 'eye' and to calculate a value for k, as before. In Figure 4.4 the line has been drawn and yields a y-axis intercept of 31.5 μg/ml. A value of k can now be determined.

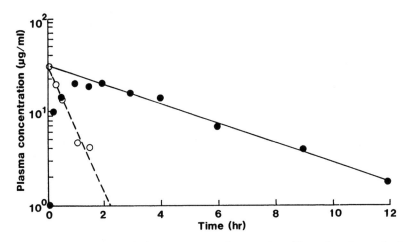

Figure 4.4 Semi-log plot of plasma concentration vs. time illustrating the method of residuals. The C^{late} line (solid line) is drawn through the terminal data points (closed circles) and the residual line (dashed line) is drawn through the calculated residuals (open circles)

$$\text{Slope} \quad = \quad \frac{\log(1.7) - \log(31.5)}{12 - 0} \quad = \quad -\frac{k}{2.3}$$

$$= \quad -\frac{1.27}{12} \quad = \quad -\frac{k}{2.3}$$

$$\text{Thus } k \quad = \quad 0.106 \times 2.3$$
$$= \quad 0.243 \text{ h}^{-1}$$

We now have a value for the intercept, A', and the slower rate constant, usually k. The next step is to determine k_a, or the faster of the two rate constants. This is where we calculate the 'residual' term. Once we have determined k we can now calculate values for the expression $\exp(-k.t)$ for early time points. If we subtract these calculated values from the actual measured data points we are determining the residuals.

$$\text{Residual} = A'.e^{-k.t} - C_{\text{measured}} \tag{4.5}$$

Since $C = A'.e^{-k.t} - A'.e^{-k_a.t}$

$$\text{Residual} = A'.e^{-k_a.t}$$

The data in Table 4.4 can be expanded to include the residual, as in Table 4.5.

Since the equation for the residual term is monoexponential in k_a it should also give a straight line on semilog graph paper. The residual values

74

Table 4.5

Time (h)	Measured C (μg/ml)	$A'.e^{-k.t}$ (μg/ml)	Residual (μg/ml)
0.0	0.0	31.5	31.5
0.25	9.6	29.6	20.0
0.50	13.8	27.9	14.1
1.0	19.9	24.7	4.8
1.5	17.7	21.9	4.2
2.0	19.8	19.4	–

are also plotted on Figure 4.4. A straight line has been drawn through the first three points to give a y-axis intercept value of 30.7 μg/ml, essentially the same as A' calculated from the C_{late} line. As before it is possible to calculate k_a from the slope of the residual line.

$$\text{Slope} = \frac{\log(30.7) - \log(5.4)}{1 - 0} = -\frac{k_a}{2.3}$$

$$= -0.755$$

$$\text{Thus } k_a = 1.74 \text{ h}^{-1}$$

As a final step in the analysis we can calculate the ratio V/F from the intercept value A'.

$$A' = \frac{F.\text{DOSE}.k_a}{V.(k_a - k)}$$

$$\frac{V}{F} = \frac{\text{DOSE}.k_a}{A'.(k_a - k)}$$

$$= \frac{500 \times 1.74}{30.7 \times (1.74 - 0.243)}$$

$$= 18.9 \text{ l}$$

For this method to work we must assume that k_a and k are different in value. In practice, a k_a/k ratio of at least five is necessary for accurate values of these two rate constants. In general, we must also assume that k_a is greater than k in order that both these parameters are separately identified. For any given set of data it is possible for the reverse to occur, i.e. that the elimination process is faster than absorption. Finally, both processes must be first-order for this technique to give accurate results. If all these assumptions are valid the method of residuals is a useful method for analysing one-compartment data collected after oral or other forms of extravascular administration.

Method of 'Wagner and Nelson' – Another approach to analysing plasma concentration vs. time data after oral administration is the method of Wagner and Nelson (1963, 1964). For this method to be applied, an estimate of the elimination rate constant is necessary. It is ideal if this has been determined previously in the same patients after a rapid intravenous dose of the drug. However, an estimate of this value can be obtained from the terminal part of the plasma concentration vs. time curve after oral or extravascular administration if the elimination rate process is slower than the absorption rate process. No other assumption need be made about the absorption process for the Wagner–Nelson method to be applicable. In fact the technique can be usefully employed to investigate the absorption process in detail. For some solid dosage forms the absorption process may involve a series of first-order dissolution and diffusion processes, or even zero-order processes. By appropriate application of the Wagner--Nelson method it is possible to learn more about the absorption step(s). For this method to apply the only assumptions needed are that the body behaves as a single homogenous compartment, and that the elimination process is first-order. The working equations can be developed by considering the mass balance equation after an oral or other extravascular dose has been given:

$$\text{Amount absorbed} \quad = \quad \text{Amount in body} + \text{Amount eliminated}$$

$$A \quad = \quad B + E$$

If we take the derivative with respect to time:

$$\frac{dA}{dt} = \frac{dB}{dt} + \frac{dE}{dt}$$

However, $B = V.C$

and

$$\frac{dB}{dt} = V. \frac{dC}{dt}$$

$$\frac{dE}{dt} = k.B$$

$$= k.V.C$$

Therefore

$$\frac{dA}{dt} = V. \frac{dC}{dt} + k.V.C$$

Integrating from $t = 0$ to $t = t$ gives:

$$_0\int^t dA = V._0\int^t dC + k.V._0\int^t C.dt$$

$$A_t = V.C_t + k.V._0\int^t C.dt \tag{4.5}$$

Dividing both sides by V gives:

$$\frac{A_t}{V} = C_t + k._0\int^t C.dt$$

where A_t/V is the amount of drug absorbed up to time t divided by the apparent volume of distribution, C_t is the plasma concentration at time t, and $_0\int^t C.dt$ is the area under the plasma concentration vs. time curve from zero time up to time t.

The above derivation can be extended to time equals infinity. Since C_t is now zero the equation becomes:

$$\frac{A_{max}}{V} = k._0\int^\infty C.dt \tag{4.6}$$

where A_{max}/V is the total amount of drug absorbed from the dosage form divided by the apparent volume of distribution and $_0\int^\infty C.dt$ is the area under the entire plasma concentration vs. time curve. Equation 4.6 can be used to compare the total amount of a dosage form which is absorbed or the bioavailability of the dosage form, as we will discuss later.

If we combine these two Equations (4.5 and 4.6) by subtracting the amount absorbed up to time t, from the total amount absorbed from the dosage form (divided by V), we obtain the term amount remaining to be absorbed $(A_{max}/V - A_t/V)$. With this term it is possible to investigate the absorption process more completely and to calculate an accurate value for the absorption rate constant. If a semilog plot of $(A_{max}/V - A_t/V)$ vs. time gives a straight line this would indicate that the absorption process can be described as first-order and a value for the absorption rate constant can be determined from the slope of the semilog plot. A straight line plot on regular graph paper would suggest that the absorption process is zero-order and the zero rate constant could be determined from the slope of the linear plot.

As an example we could consider the data given above in Table 4.5. When performing the Wagner–Nelson calculation manually it is often helpful to set up the various terms in a tabular form (Table 4.6).

A plot of the results in column 6 of Table 4.6 on semilog graph paper should now give a straight line with a slope of $k_a/2.3$.

Table 4.6

Time (h)	C (μg/ml)	$_0\int{}^tC.dt$	$k._0\int{}^t C.dt$	At/V	$(A_{max}/V - At/V)$
0.0	0.0	0.0	0.0	0.0	26.7
0.25	9.6	1.2	0.3	9.9	16.8
0.5	13.8	4.1	1.0	14.8	11.9
1.0	19.9	12.6	2.9	22.8	3.8
1.5	17.7	22.0	5.1	22.8	3.8
2.0	19.8	31.3	7.3	27.1	–
3.0	15.4	49.0	11.4	26.8	–
4.0	13.4	63.3	14.8	28.2	–
6.0	6.5	83.2	19.5	26.0	–
9.0	3.8	98.7	23.1	26.9	–
12.0	1.7	106.9	25.0	26.7	–
inf	–	113.9	26.7	26.7	–

$$\text{Slope} = \frac{\log (26.2) - \log (1)}{2}$$

$$= -0.709$$

$$k_a = -0.709 \times (-2.3)$$

$$= 1.63 \text{ h}^{-1}$$

Non-linear regression analysis – Once the method of residuals or the Wagner–Nelson method has been used to analyse the data it may be appropriate to further refine the parameter values by non-linear regression analysis. In that case we can use the parameter values already determined as initial estimates for the non-linear fitting process. As before, the MULTI program was used to obtained 'best fit' values for the parameters k_a, k, and V/F. The program lines in Scheme 4.3 are included in the program MULTI (*see* Appendix) and used to describe the pharmacokinetic model of first-order absorption and elimination with a single central compartment.

1030 CP = (CN(1) * P(2) / (P(3) * (P(2) – P(1)))) * (EXP (–P(1) *T) – EXP (–P(2) * T)): RETURN
1031 REM P(1) = KEL:P(2) = KA:P(3) = V:CN(1) = DOSE
11630 M = 3:NC = 1:PL$(1) = "KEL":PL$(2) = "KA":PL$(3) = "V/F":CN$(1) = "DOSE":MD$ = "ONE COMPARTMENT-ORAL": GOTO 11700

Scheme 4.3

When the data were weighted by each value squared, the parameter values were: k, 0.243 h^{-1}; k_a, 1.70 h^{-1}; and V/F, 18.4 l. The parameter values obtained when each data point was weighted equally were: k, 0.244 h^{-1}; k_a, 1.60 h^{-1}; and V/F, 18.0 l. The r^2 values were 0.982 and 1.00 for the unweighted and weighted fittings, respectively.

Bioavailability, F

In the previous section, methods for determining a value for the rate of absorption were described. The value of this parameter, k_a, only describes part of the situation. The extent of absorption is also an important part of the overall performance of an oral dosage form. The extent of absorption, or bioavailability (F) is defined as the fraction of the administered dose which is delivered to the general circulation of the patient. Impediments to total absorption include poor dosage form, metabolism or degradation of the drug in the gastrointestinal tract, and extensive metabolism of the drug in the liver ('first-pass effect'). The effect of all these processes are included in the parameter F. Ideally an absolute bioavailability value is determined which takes into account all the possibilities for reduced absorption. The absolute bioavailability is most easily determined by comparing the dosage form of interest with an intravenously administered dose of the same drug. An alternative approach is to determine a relative bioavailability. Most commonly this is determined by comparing one dosage form with an orally administered solution of the drug or with another 'reference' dosage form. In this case it is not possible to take into account some of the factors which cause a reduction in bioavailability, hence the designation *relative bioavailability*.

Area under the plasma vs. time curve comparisons – In a previous section we derived Equation 4.6 for the maximum amount of a drug absorbed after oral administration (A_{max}) divided by the apparent volume of distribution (V). For an oral dose the maximum amount absorbed is equal to the dose multiplied by the bioavailability. Thus,

$$\text{DOSE}_{oral}.F_{oral} = A_{max} = k.V.\text{AUC}_{oral} \qquad (4.7)$$

or

$$F_{oral} = \frac{k.V.\text{AUC}_{oral}}{\text{DOSE}_{oral}} \qquad (4.8)$$

The relative bioavailability of one oral dosage can be compared with the bioavailability of another, by comparing the AUC values determined after administration of each dosage form to a panel of subjects. The relative bioavailability, F, can be calculated from the ratio F_1/F_2, thus:

$$F = \frac{F_1}{F_2} = \frac{k_1.V_1.\text{AUC}_1.\text{DOSE}_2}{k_2.V_2.\text{AUC}_2.\text{DOSE}_1} \qquad (4.9)$$

If we assume that k and V are unchanged from one dosage administration to another, and if the same dose is given this equation simplifies to a comparison of AUC values alone.

$$F \;=\; \frac{AUC_1}{AUC_2} \tag{4.10}$$

As an example, if the AUC measured after a test dosage form was 114 μg h ml^{-1} and after the standard dosage form the AUC value was 125 μg h ml^{-1}, the relative bioavailability of the test dosage form is simply 114/125, i.e. 0.91 or 91%.

The absolute bioavailability of the test dosage form can be determined if we can measure an AUC value after intravenous administration of the drug. From the equations presented above we can equate the i.v. dose with $k.V.AUC_{IV}$.

Thus,

$$F \;=\; \frac{F_{oral}}{F_{IV}} \;=\; F_{oral}$$

since $F_{IV} = 1$.

Therefore,

$$F \;=\; \frac{k_{oral}.V_{oral}.AUC_{oral}.DOSE_{IV}}{k_{IV}.V_{IV}.AUC_{IV}.DOSE_{oral}} \tag{4.11}$$

Again if we assume that k and V do not change from one dose administration to another, and if we give the same dose on each occasion, this equation for F simplifies to a comparison of AUC values.

$$F \;=\; \frac{AUC_{oral}}{AUC_{IV}} \tag{4.12}$$

As an example, if an oral dosage form gave an AUC value calculated by the trapezoidal rule of 114 μg h ml^{-1} and an intravenous injection containing the same dose of drug produced an AUC value of 130 μg h ml^{-1}, the absolute bioavailability of the test dosage form can be calculated as 114/130, i.e. 0.88 or 88%.

Non-linear regression analysis – In the determination of k_a by non-linear regression analysis, the term V/F was also determined. A value for the apparent volume of distribution can often be determined independently. For example, after intravenous administration of the drug, a value for V may be determined by non-linear regression analysis of the resultant plasma concentration vs. time data. It is now a simple matter to calculate the bioavailability of the oral dosage form.

$$F \;=\; \frac{V_{IV}}{(V/F)_{oral}}$$

As an example, if the V/F value after an oral dosage form was found to be 18 l and the V value determined after an intravenous administration was 15 l, the bioavailability of the oral dosage form could be calculated as 15/18, i.e. 0.83 or 83%.

One-compartment pharmacokinetic model with Michaelis–Menten elimination kinetics

For some drugs evidence of non-linear elimination kinetics is obvious at therapeutically useful plasma concentration levels. For these drugs, inclusion of Michaelis–Menten kinetics into the pharmacokinetic model may be necessary. It is usually difficult to determine accurate values for the Michaelis–Menten parameters from a single drug administration. A wide range in plasma concentrations is necessary for a thorough and accurate pharmacokinetic analysis. For most drugs which exhibit Michaelis–Menten kinetics this would entail high, possibly toxic concentrations, or quite low, subtherapeutic concentrations. It is therefore highly unlikely that the Michaelis–Menten parameters could be determined accurately after a single drug administration to a patient. However, if the drug can be given as a multiple dose regimen it is possible to determine some information about the Michaelis–Menten parameters. It can be shown that the plateau or steady state plasma concentration can be related to the dosing rate, and the Michaelis–Menten parameters V_m and K_m.

$$R = \frac{V_m . C_{ss}}{K_m + C_{ss}} \tag{4.13}$$

or

$$C_{ss} = \frac{K_m . R}{V_m - R} \tag{4.14}$$

where R is the dosing rate, dose per day or per hour. For example if V_m is 500 mg/day and K_m is 5 mg/l a dosing rate of 300 mg per day (150 mg every 12 h or 300 mg, once a day) would produce a steady state plasma concentration of 7.5 mg/l. These equations could also be used to calculate an appropriate dosing rate if the Michaelis–Menten parameters were known. With two unknowns it is necessary to make at least two determinations of C_{ss} after two different dosing rates. Alternatively, if an average value could be assumed for one of the Michaelis–Menten parameters the other could be determined after one multiple dose regimen. In practice, the results from one dosing regimen can be used to make an appropriate adjustment in the dosing rate. With a second steady state plasma concentration both parameter values can be estimated for a further refinement in the dosing regimen, if appropriate.

As an example we could consider a patient given 300 mg of drug per day for a number of weeks. If the steady state plasma concentration was then determined to be 10 mg/l and if we know that the average V_m value is 600 mg/day it is possible to estimate K_m as 10 mg/l. We could use this information to calculate an appropriate dosing rate to produce a steady state plasma concentration of 15 mg/l. If V_m is 600 mg per day in this patient we could expect that a dosing rate of 360 mg per day would produce a steady state plasma concentration of 15 mg/l. (It should be noted that if V_m was actually 400 mg/day the K_m value would be 3.3 mg/l and the projected steady state plasma concentration on this dosing regimen would now be 20 mg/l.) If the steady state plasma concentration measured after the second, 360 mg per day, dosing regimen was actually 18 mg/l both K_m and V_m can be calculated for a further dosing regimen adjustment.

Therefore with these data:

R_1 = 300 mg per day; $C_{ss,1}$ = 10 mg/l

and

R_2 = 360 mg per day; $C_{ss,2}$ = 18 mg/l

values for K_m and V_m can be calculated by solving simultaneous equations. The values thereby obtained are K_m = 6 mg/l and V_m = 480 mg/day.

TWO-COMPARTMENT PHARMACOKINETIC MODEL

I.V. bolus

Often plasma concentration vs. time data collected after a rapid i.v. injection appear to be biexponential. That is, the data plotted on semilog graph paper appear to follow two separate lines, a rapid α phase and a slower terminal β phase. The term biexponential means that the curve can be described by an equation with two exponential terms.

$$C = A.\exp^{-\alpha.t} + B.\exp^{-\beta.t} \qquad (4.15)$$

This equation is similar to Equation 4.3 described above; in that case the second exponential term was due to absorption. As before the method of residuals or non-linear regression analysis can be used to calculate 'best fit' values for the parameters A, B, α and β. These values, in turn, can be used to calculate the values of the two-compartment parameters, k_{12}, k_{21}, k_{10}, and V_1 described in Figure 3.9, using Equations 3.21–3.24.

As an example, data were calculated with the parameter values dose = 250 mg, A = 20 μg/ml, B = 4 μg/ml, α = 1.5 h^{-1}, and β = 0.07 h^{-1}. These values correspond to the parameter values, k_{10} = 0.340 h^{-1}, k_{12} = 0.921 h^{-1}, k_{21} = 0.308 h^{-1}, and V_1 = 10.4 l. As before, 10% random error proportional to the calculated plasma concentration was added to each data point (Table 4.7).

Table 4.7

Time (h)	Plasma concentration (μg/ml)
0.083	22.02
0.167	19.41
0.25	17.73
0.50	13.52
0.75	10.69
1.0	9.52
1.5	5.79
2.0	3.64
4.0	3.15
6.0	2.42
8.0	2.33
12.0	1.49

If the data are plotted on semilog graph paper as in Figure 4.5, the biexponential nature of the data is clear. By 'eye' or by linear regression analysis it is possible to draw a line through the terminal data points. From this line values for B and β can be calculated as 4.38 μg/ml and 0.0879 h^{-1}, respectively. The residual line can be calculated by subtracting the extension of the terminal line and the early data points. Again a reasonably straight line results on semilog graph paper. From the residual line, values of A and α can be calculated as 19.9 μg/ml and 1.47 h^{-1}, respectively. From these values the parameters k_{10}, k_{12}, k_{21}, and V_1 can be calculated as 0.384 h^{-1}, 0.841 h^{-1}, 0.338 h^{-1}, and 10.3 l, respectively. As described above, the method of residuals can give accurate values only if the ratio of α/β is greater than 5. In the present example α/β can be calculated as 16.7; therefore we can expect that the parameter values are reasonably accurate.

Finally the MULTI program can be used to obtain a non-linear fit to the plasma concentration vs. time data. Using the initial parameter values calculated above and two weighting schemes (equal weight and weight inversely proportional to each value squared) the data were fitted to the two-compartment pharmacokinetic model described by the program lines (*see* Appendix for the rest of the program MULTI) in Scheme 4.4.

```
1040 CP = P(1) * EXP (−P(2) * T) + P(3) * EXP (−P(4) * T): RETURN
1041 REM P(1) = A:P(2) = ALPHA:P(3) = B:P(4) = BETA
11640 M = 4:NC = 0:PL$(1) = "A":PL$(2) = "ALPHA":PL$(3) =
      "B":PL$(4) = "BETA":MD$ = "TWO COMPARTMENT-I.V.
      BOLUS": GOTO 11700
```

Scheme 4.4

With the equal weighting scheme the 'best fit' parameter values were k_{10} = 0.300 h^{-1}, k_{12} = 0.835 h^{-1}, k_{21} = 0.258 h^{-1}, and V_1 = 11.6 l, whereas with the proportional weighting scheme the parameter values were k_{10} =

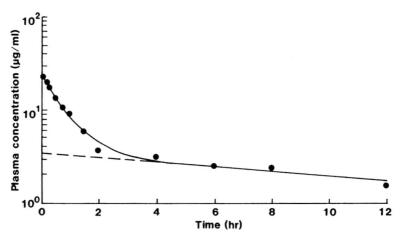

Figure 4.5 Semilogarithmic plot of plasma concentration vs. time. The best fit line (solid line) to the two-compartment model is drawn through the data points (closed circles). The dashed line is drawn through the terminal points and extrapolated back to the y-axis to give a value for B.

0.352 h^{-1}, k_{12} = 0.919 h^{-1}, k_{21} = 0.320 h^{-1}, V_1 = 11.2 l. For this example the proportional weighting scheme gave the more accurate parameter values. The r^2 values were 0.997 and 1.000, respectively, for the weighted and unweighted fit to the data.

Oral administration

For a drug following two-compartment pharmacokinetics the plasma concentration vs. time data after oral administration will follow a triexponential equation. The three exponential terms are α, β, and k_a. Often, however, it is not possible to determine accurate values for these parameters using the method of residuals unless there is a wide variation between each of the parameters. A ratio of at least 5 between each rate constant is necessary to enable successful resolution of all the exponential terms with the method of residuals. It is also difficult to use non-linear regression analysis. For this method to be successful there needs to be a good separation in the values of the three parameters and sufficient data points. However, if parameter values for the drug can be determined after intravenous administration, as well as after oral administration, a deconvolution technique can be used to determine the absorption characteristics of the dosage form. One such method is that of Loo and Riegelman (1968). This method mathematically subtracts the distribution and elimination kinetics (derived from the intravenous data) from the oral data, leaving information about the absorption rate constant (k_a). The extent of absorption can be determined as before by comparing the area under the plasma concentration vs. time curve obtained after oral administration with the curve obtained after intravenous administration.

References

Wagner, J.G. and Nelson, E. (1963). *J. Pharm. Sci.*, **52**, 610–11
Wagner, J.G. and Nelson, E. (1964). *J. Pharm. Sci.*, **53**, 1392–1403
Loo, J.C.K. and Riegelman, S. (1968). *J. Pharm. Sci.*, **57**, 918–28

5
Pharmacokinetic parameters and their implications in health and disease

As explained in earlier chapters, a number of pharmacokinetic parameters may be calculated for a drug given to a patient. Parameters relating to drug absorption (drug entry into the body – sometimes called drug invasion) may vary in magnitude with the route of drug administration, whereas the values of those relating to drug distribution and elimination (i.e. drug disposition) apply irrespective of how the drug is administered. In this chapter the individual pharmacokinetic parameters are considered in turn, and their derivations, their reliability and the deductions that may justifiably be drawn from them in the healthy and diseased state are discussed.

PARAMETERS RELATING TO DRUG DISPOSITION

The fraction of the drug dose excreted unchanged

Although this parameter is not always quoted in pharmacokinetic work, knowledge of its value is essential in thinking about the elimination of a given drug. For most drugs the great majority of the unmetabolized molecules of the drug are excreted in urine; however, for volatile substances (such as the gaseous anaesthetics) expired air may be the main route of excretion. Excluding the gaseous anaesthetics, in nearly all instances the fraction of drug dose excreted unchanged by routes other than urine (e.g. tears, sweat, breast milk, faeces) is small, and often negligible. Assuming that the whole of a given dose of drug has entered the body (as must be the case with intravenous or intramuscular administration of the drug), the fraction of the drug dose that has not been excreted unchanged represents the portion of the drug dose eliminated by metabolism (biotransformation).

Thus the fraction excreted unchanged in urine, the $fe(\infty)$, measured by specific assay and preferably after intravenous administration of a known drug dose, indicates the extent to which the drug is eliminated by excretion unchanged, and, by difference, the extent to which it is eliminated by metabolism. This knowledge is a prerequisite for interpreting clearance values (see below).

Work with radioactive-labelled drugs can easily produce confusing information in relation to the parameter $fe(\infty)$. This can happen if the 'label' remains on metabolites produced by biotransformation of the parent drug, and whole urine radioactivity is measured without a preliminary separation procedure to isolate parent substance from metabolites. Accurate values for the parameter $fe(\infty)$ depend on complete urine collection for a long enough time for all, or nearly all, of the drug dose given to be eliminated. This can be ascertained by determining that the drug concentration has become unmeasurable in plasma. As a rough guide, urine collection should continue for some seven terminal halflives of the drug. There can be major practical problems in collecting all urine passed over so long a period, because of the risk of accidental loss of specimens.

If a drug is eliminated chiefly by renal execution in unmetabolized form (i.e. its $fe(\infty)$ is>0.5), any decrease in renal function, as occurs with ageing and various forms of renal (glomerular) disease, e.g. nephritis, may make a reduction necessary in the drug dose required to provide a given pharmacological effect. For drugs for which the only substantial route of elimination is by renal mechanisms (i.e. a $fe(\infty)$>0.75 or 0.80) it may be possible to correlate the necessary drug dosage reduction in renal disease with measures of renal function, e.g. the creatinine clearance. Such is the case for digoxin, for example. For such drugs, it may often be unnecessary to modify dosages in the presence of decreased liver function. The converse would tend to apply for drugs for which the fraction excreted unchanged was low. Dosage of these drugs may need to be reduced if liver function was decreased, but would not need to be reduced if renal function was diminished.

Fraction of the drug in plasma bound to plasma proteins

Figures are widely available for the proportions of the molecules of various drugs that exist in plasma bound to plasma proteins. It is the unbound (free) drug in plasma that equilibrates with drug in the extravascular compartment and in the biophase. Therefore, knowledge of free drug concentration is clearly clinically relevant. However, because drug binding to plasma proteins is nearly always readily reversible, concentration of drug bound to plasma proteins, concentration of drug in plasma water and extravascular drug concentration tend to vary in parallel. There is a finite number of drug binding sites available on plasma proteins. Therefore, drug binding to plasma proteins is in its nature a saturable process that will follow non-linear behavioural characteristics. In practice it appears uncommon for plasma protein binding capacity to approach saturation at concentrations of drugs that apply therapeutically, but occasionally such a situation may occur. This simply means that one usually happens to work in a pseudo-linear phase of the fundamentally non-linear relation between free and

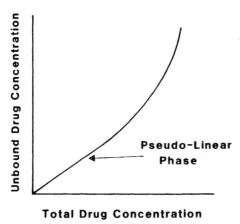

Figure 5.1 Relationship between concentrations of unbound and bound plus unbound drug in plasma

total drug in plasma (Figure 5.1). Matters are simplified when it has been shown experimentally that the relation between protein-bound and protein-unbound drug in plasma is reasonably constant over the concentration range in which one is interested. If the relationship between the two changes, so that the binding capacity appears to approach saturation as total plasma drug concentration rises, certain difficulties appear:

(1) Since the relation between unbound ('free') drug concentration and total drug concentration in plasma is as shown in Figure 5.1, a constancy of relation between whole plasma drug concentration and biological effect (which is proportionate to 'free' drug) may not apply. In such circumstances it will be more meaningful to measure drug concentrations in plasma water, i.e. 'free' drug.

(2) At higher plasma total drug concentrations, the disproportionate increase in unbound drug relative to total drug means that more drug than might have been anticipated is available for elimination and for transfer to the extravascular compartment (where one almost always has no direct information as to the relationship between drug free in extravascular water and drug bound to various tissue molecules). Clearance will tend to increase as plasma total drug concentration rises; it may increasingly be invalid to calculate elimination rate constants from total plasma drug concentration vs. time data, because elimination kinetics will in these circumstances appear not to follow simple exponential processes. These departures from linearity might suggest that the plasma concentration vs. time curve would better be expressed in terms of plasma water drug concentrations. However, this would lead to values for certain pharmacokinetic parameters which would also be expressed on an

unfamiliar basis, i.e. plasma water rather than whole plasma drug concentrations. While the actual physical volumes of plasma water and whole plasma would be virtually identical, the values of pharmacokinetic parameters expressed in terms of these different bases could show major differences if a significant fraction of the drug in plasma was protein bound.

One may be able to predict trends which could arise from this source of non-linearity in pharmacokinetics. However, it will often be impossible to anticipate the actual magnitude of the changes because one will necessarily be ignorant of what will happen simultaneously to drug concentrations in the aqueous element of the extravascular compartment, with its unknown numbers of drug binding sites.

Plasma protein binding of drugs may change in physiological states (e.g. later pregnancy, old age), in disease, and when other drugs are administered which affect the binding of the drug in question. Disease (mainly hepatic and renal disease) may reduce plasma protein binding of a drug either because of qualitative or quantitative changes in the plasma proteins synthesized, because of loss of plasma protein (as in the nephrotic syndrome), or because disease causes accumulation of endogenous substances which may affect the drug binding capacity of the plasma proteins, e.g. endogenous acids in uraemia. While such alterations in plasma protein binding capacity have implications for pharmacokinetics, and much has been written on them, the results of such changes in binding have often not proved of great magnitude. This is possibly so because the alterations only occur in the vascular compartment, and for many drugs this may be only a small component of the total apparent volume of drug distribution. Extravascular events, which cannot be predicted with any reasonable security in the present state of knowledge, may largely buffer the effects on various pharmacokinetic parameters of any changes that occur in plasma as a result of altered plasma protein binding of drugs.

The plasma protein binding of a drug may be measured directly in plasma samples, usually by equilibrium dialysis or ultrafiltration techniques, carried out at 37 °C. Alternatively, plasma protein binding may be estimated indirectly by measuring drug concentrations in biological fluids which have low protein contents relative to plasma. Thus one may measure drug concentration in saliva (with allowance being made for the differences in pH between plasma and saliva causing differences in ionization of the drug in the two fluids, since only non-ionized drug molecules will equilibrate between the two fluids). Another possibility is to measure drug in CSF (remembering that certain organic acids are actively extruded from CSF by choroid plexus cells). Results from such indirect methods should be accepted for a given drug only after values obtained by these methods have been shown experimentally to correlate with direct measurements of its plasma protein binding.

The main plasma protein to which both anionic (acid) and cationic (basic) drugs bind is albumin. However, many basic drugs also bind to α_1-acid glycoprotein, and occasionally drugs bind to specific protein fractions, e.g. adrenal glucocorticoids to particular globulins. Plasma albumin concentrations tend to decline in the aged, and are reduced in various forms of hepatocellular disease, malnutrition and the nephrotic syndrome. In these circumstances the plasma protein binding of many drugs will be reduced, and there will be more free drug relative to total drug concentration than in normal persons. Some of the increased amounts of free drug will be cleared by metabolism or by being excreted unchanged. Some will be distributed through the extravascular compartment. In general the greater the apparent volume of distribution of a drug, the more this latter effect will 'buffer' the effect of a reduced plasma protein binding capacity. However, the uncertain element in this situation is the extent to which tissue protein binding capacity may be altered by the disease state. Little information is available on this matter. It is, therefore, difficult to predict the effects of measured alterations in plasma protein binding capacity for drugs based on the values of other pharmacokinetic parameters in various physiological and diseased states.

The halflife

The halflife ($t_{\frac{1}{2}}$) or more exactly, the terminal halflife of the drug in plasma ($t_{\frac{1}{2},z}$), is derived from the rate constant k, or β.

If the term 'halflife' is used without qualification, it is generally taken to refer to the plasma halflife of a drug. The halflife ($t_{\frac{1}{2}}$) is a measure of the terminal rate of decline of drug concentration in plasma. It is calculated through the following relationship:

$$t_{\frac{1}{2}} = \ln2/\text{rate constant of decline} = 0.693/\text{rate constant of decline} = 0.693/k$$
$$\text{or } 0.693/\beta$$

In the case of a one-compartment pharmacokinetic model, where the drug behaves as if almost instantaneously distributed throughout that portion of the body into which it can enter, the rate constant of plasma level decline for calculating $t_{\frac{1}{2}}$ is the elimination rate constant (k) itself. In the case of a multicompartment model, the relevant rate constant is the hybrid rate constant (β) which refers to the terminal rate of decline in plasma drug concentration. The derivation of β is shown in Chapter 3. In practice β is calculated fairly simply from mathematical analysis of the terminal stage of the plasma drug level vs. time curve. In the case of a multicompartment model the terminal halflife is not purely an elimination halflife from any particular compartment. It is simply a halflife of decline in plasma drug concentration, and reflects the effects of intercompartmental drug transfers as well as overall elimination. The relevant rate constants are a little easier to use than the corresponding halflives in calculating other pharmacokinetic parameters. However, clinicians generally find it simpler to think in terms of hours, or minutes (the units of halflife), than in terms of fractions per hour (the unit of rate constants). Therefore the halflife rather than the rate constant will be the parameter discussed in the following subsections.

Reliability of estimation of halflife values

The terminal halflife of a drug is measured in the later phase of decline of plasma drug concentrations, after the dose of the drug studied has achieved its definitive distributional equilibria throughout the body. By this stage plasma drug concentrations may be relatively low, and they will decline further with time. Therefore, assay error on plasma collected at these times is likely to be of greater relative magnitude than on samples collected earlier in the plasma concentration vs. time course of the drug, when concentrations are higher. If the assay used is not sufficiently sensitive, drug concentrations in the true terminal elimination phase may not be measurable, or may not be able to be studied for long enough for the terminal phase to be distinguished from an earlier phase of drug disposition. The shorter the halflife appears to be, when working near the limit of assay sensitivity, the greater the chance that the true terminal halflife stage may not have been studied in full, and that the halflife as determined may have been based on a mixture of α and β phases of plasma level decline. If the assay used is not specific for the drug itself, failing to distinguish between it and its metabolites, there is the obvious possibility that the halflife determined will be that of drug plus metabolites, and thus may not be a true value for the drug itself. Also, in the later phase of the plasma level vs. time curve, when terminal halflife values should be determined, drugs which are in reality eliminated dominantly by processes which follow Michaelis–Menten kinetics are approaching the limiting circumstance $(K_m >> C_t)$ where exponential kinetics will also provide a very good fit to the plasma level vs. time data. Hence a drug which, strictly speaking, does not have a halflife because its elimination does not follow an exponential process, can have a halflife measured, apparently with very satisfactory accuracy. If this halflife value is used to draw conclusions about the drug at higher concentrations, major and sometimes dangerous errors may arise, since deductions will have been based on kinetics that are not valid over a wide enough concentration range.

The anticonvulsant, phenytoin, provides an example of this phenomenon. Measurements of the K_m values of this drug in humans indicate that its elimination capacity becomes half-saturated at plasma concentrations of around 4–6 mg/l. Plasma drug concentrations of 10–20 mg/l usually provide the optimal compromise between control of epilepsy and adverse effects of therapy. After single oral doses of phenytoin, which may produce plasma drug levels in this 'therapeutic' range, conventional linear pharmacokinetic analysis can provide apparently precise halflife values of $20 \pm$ S.D. 9 h (Arnold and Gerber, 1970), corresponding to a mean k value of 0.0346 h^{-1}. However, if this value is used (rather than the V_{max} and K_m values, which are a good deal more difficult to compute) in predicting plasma drug levels and their time courses produced by increased phenytoin doses, serious underestimations are likely once plasma phenytoin levels are in the therapeutic range. Phenytoin intoxication may easily be produced.

Elimination halflives of a drug in the normal population may show considerable interindividual variation so that there are obvious dangers in applying population mean values to guide the therapy of individual patients. Published halflife values have often been determined after the first dose of a drug is given to healthy volunteers. Age and sex, disease, concurrent intake of other drugs and continued use of the drug in question may all influence its elimination rate. Therefore, published tables of halflife values, and ranges of values, sometimes constitute a rather insecure basis for taking therapeutic decisions for individual patients who receive a drug, often in long-term therapy. Despite these reservations, in practice halflife values, if employed cautiously, often prove a very useful guide to drug treatment.

Depending on whether a drug is cleared predominantly by renal excretion unchanged (high $fe(\infty)$ value) or by metabolism (low $fe(\infty)$ value) its halflife may change in the presence of various physiological and pathological circumstances. For drugs cleared by renal excretory mechanisms, halflives tend to be prolonged in the very young infant, in the elderly and in those with renal disease (particularly glomerular disease), and halflives tend to be shortened in pregnancy (where glomerular filtration rate is high). For drugs cleared by metabolism the halflife tends to be somewhat prolonged in the very young and the old, and is likely to be increased in liver cell disease, e.g. hepatitis, cirrhosis; at least for some such drugs the halflife may be shortened in pregnancy. However, in these circumstances one is not necessarily entitled to deduce that drug dose should be altered reciprocally to halflife change to maintain the desired therapeutic effects. Halflife measures a rate of change in the plasma drug level, not the amount of drug elimination. The more appropriate parameter on which therapeutic decisions should be based is the clearance (CL), as will be discussed later.

Implications of the halflife

Much clinical pharmacokinetic thinking revolves around the relation between pharmacological effects and drug concentrations in plasma. The halflife allows one to draw a number of valid conclusions regarding the time course of plasma drug concentration, so long as one is dealing with a drug that is eliminated by processes that follow linear kinetics over the concentration range under consideration. Renal excretion mechanisms are generally dependent on passive transfer processes, so that drugs cleared predominantly by renal mechanisms generally follow linear elimination kinetics. Drugs cleared by metabolism are more likely to show departures from linearity in their kinetics, since metabolic capacity can become saturated.

The time course of the decline in plasma drug concentration – Over each halflife plasma drug concentration falls to 50% of its value at the start of the halflife interval under scrutiny. Parallel changes in drug concentration throughout the body would be expected. Thus after two consecutive halflives plasma drug levels are 25% of their initial value, after three halflives 12.5%, after four halflives 6.25%, after five halflives 3.13%, after six halflives 1.57% and after seven halflives, 0.79%. Although in theory plasma drug concentrations never become zero with an exponential process of n practical terms the amount of drug remaining in the body always have become negligible by the expiry of four or five e halflives.

Time to achieve a steady state (T_{ss}) – With repeated doses of a drug at regular intervals, each dose being given before all the drug from the previous dose has been eliminated, mean plasma drug concentration during each dosage interval rises. The rise continues till mean plasma drug concentration reaches a plateau, when the amount of drug entering the body during each dosage interval equals the amount of drug eliminated in the same period. This situation is referred to as the 'steady state'. In the steady state, plasma drug concentration is not constant from moment to moment over the duration of each dosage interval. Particularly with rapidly absorbed and rapidly eliminated drugs, there may be substantial rises and then falls in plasma drug level during each dosage interval under steady state conditions. However, the mean plasma level is constant from one dosage interval to the next.

From the clinician's point of view, the time to achieve steady state conditions defines the shortest time for the maximum (both beneficial and adverse) effects of the drug dose he has prescribed to occur. It is often very valuable to know this time. If dosage is increased before enough time has passed for a lower dose to have achieved steady state plasma levels there is a significantly increased chance of producing subsequent overdosage manifestations and of using an unnecessarily high drug dosage. A drug will achieve 50% of its steady state mean plasma levels after one halflife, 75% of the levels after two halflives, 88% of the levels after three halflives, 94% of the levels after four halflives and 97% of the mean steady state levels by the expiry of five halflives. For most clinical purposes it suffices to accept that a steady state regarding the drug in question will be achieved in four to five halflives. Should the halflife shorten with repeated intake of a drug, because its elimination rate increases with continued exposure to the drug (autoinduction of metabolism), the steady state may occur earlier than expected.

The area under the plasma level vs. time curve (AUC)

As displayed on a graphical plot after a dose of a drug, the area under the plasma concentration vs. time curve (the AUC), extended to infinity, represents a result of the drug's entry into the body, of its distribution around the body, and of its elimination from that body. The $AUC_{0\rightarrow\infty}$ is thus a function of the drug dose entering the circulation, and of the drug's absorption, distribution and elimination in the body under consideration. The unit of AUC is concentration×time, e.g. mg l^{-1} h. The value of the AUC depends on many factors in the individual, as well as on the drug's own inherent properties and the drug dose. Because AUC values are determined by so many individual variables, the AUC is usually not a quoted pharmacokinetic parameter for a given drug. However, the AUC value in the individual is used to derive other pharmacokinetic parameters which are not as susceptible to individual variations. Only if the amount of drug entering the circulation, and its absorption, distribution and elimination remain constant for a given drug in an individual from time to time, and if his personal anatomy and physiology remain unaltered, should the AUC remain constant for that individual.

AUC may be calculated in several ways. The area may be measured by (1) planimetry carried out on a plot of the plasma concentration vs. time curve, (2) cutting out and weighing the whole area of graph paper under the curve, and also, for calibration purposes, a portion of the sheet of paper of known dimensions (i.e. known concentration×time units), (3) trapezoidal rule integration of the plasma concentration vs. time data, or (4) calculation from the parameters of the equation of best fit to the plasma concentration vs. time data. The first three approaches are usually said not to depend on assigning any particular pharmacokinetic model of drug disposition to the substance in question. However, the fourth approach requires knowledge of the most appropriate pharmacokinetic model. The first three approaches measure only $AUC_{0\to t}$, i.e. AUC from the outset to the last measured plasma concentration. To measure AUC from time t to infinity, and to then calculate $AUC_{0\to\infty}$ ($= AUC_{0\to t} + AUC_{t\to\infty}$), one must make assumptions about the shape of the (unmeasured) terminal phase of the plasma level vs. time curve. The usual assumption is that the terminal phase can be represented by a monoexponential process, in which case $AUC_{t\to\infty} = C_t/k$ or C_t/β, i.e. the value of the last data point divided by the terminal rate constant of plasma level decline. In adopting this policy one assumes linear kinetics apply, though if the value of C_t is small enough the error is likely to be negligible even if Michaelis–Menten kinetics should have been applied.

Calculation of $AUC_{0\to\infty}$ from the parameters of the equation of best fit to the plasma concentration vs. time data assumes linear pharmacokinetics, i.e. $C_t = \Sigma a_i e^{-b_i t}$. In this case $AUC_{0\to\infty} = \Sigma a_i/b_i$.

When a patient is in a steady state as regards a drug, it is obvious that he will absorb as much drug as he eliminates over each dosage interval. His plasma level vs. time curve should be identical from one dosage interval to the next. In this circumstance AUC across a dosage interval, or across 24 h, is a function of the dose (per dosage interval or per 24 h, respectively), and of the drug's absorption, distribution and elimination parameters in the individual.

The above considerations regarding AUC after a single drug dose, and in the steady state are important when the parameter is used to derive other pharmacokinetic parameters.

Clearance (CL)

The parameter clearance relates the rate of elimination of a drug to its concentration in a relevant body fluid.

$$CL = \frac{\text{rate of elimination}}{C}$$

Whole body, systemic or plasma clearance refers to the rate of elimination of a drug by all routes, relative to its concentration in plasma. Such a clearance is in some ways analogous to the parameter apparent volume of distribution (V, see below) which relates the total amount of drug in the body to its plasma concentration.

It should be noted that the clearance is not a measure of the amount of drug that is being eliminated, but of a volume of the body from which the drug is eliminated, or 'cleared', for each unit of time. However, a conceptual artifice is adopted in expressing clearance in this way. The drug is thought of as if it is completely removed from a portion of its volume of distribution in each unit of time (this rate per unit time being the clearance value) while the drug's concentration is left unaltered in the remainder of the volume of distribution. Clearance so determined has a constant value in a given patient irrespective of plasma drug concentration, so long as the drug in question follows linear pharmacokinetics. On the other hand, the rate of drug elimination (not elimination rate constant) varies with plasma drug concentration.

Clearance may be specified in terms of drug concentration in whole blood, in plasma or in plasma water (i.e. 'unbound' or 'free' drug). The concept may also be related to elimination of a drug via particular routes, or via particular organs, rather than elimination from the whole body, as discussed above. The unit of clearance, like that of flow, is volume per unit time. If a drug has a plasma clearance of 1 l/h, and a plasma concentration of 1 mg/l, 1 mg of the drug will be eliminated in the first hour under consideration.

If one considers clearance in relation to a particular route or organ of drug elimination, the so-called 'physiological approach', the following considerations apply. The rate of presentation of drug to the organ of elimination is the product of the arterial blood flow to the organ (Q) and the drug concentration in the blood entering the organ (C_A), i.e. $Q.C_A$. The rate at which drug leaves the organ is $Q.C_V$ (where C_V is drug concentration in the venous blood leaving the organ). The difference $Q.C_A - Q.C_V$ represents the rate of drug removal (or extraction by the organ). The rate of extraction divided by the rate of drug presentation to the organ defines an extraction ratio (E).

$$ E = \frac{Q.C_A - Q.C_V}{Q.C_A} = \frac{(C_A - C_V)}{C_A} $$

The value of the extraction ratio must lie between 0, when no drug is extracted by the organ, and 1, when all the drug entering the organ is extracted by it. The rate of extraction $Q.(C_A - C_V)$, divided by the incoming drug concentration (C_A), defines the clearance:

$$ CL = \frac{Q.(C_A - C_V)}{C_A} = Q.E. $$

Thus the organ clearance is simply the product of extraction ratio and organ blood flow. Should it be possible to measure the amount of drug extracted (as when a drug is excreted into urine, and the amount of drug appearing in urine is measured directly), $Q.(C_A-C_V)$ is known without measuring Q, C_A and C_V, and if mean plasma drug concentration over the time of study is accepted as a measure of C_A, clearance can be determined from the relationship above.

Properties of clearance

Clearance can be related to the eliminating organ or organs, or to the whole body, as mentioned above. One may thus speak of renal and extrarenal clearance, or renal and metabolic clearance (it being assumed that any drug not cleared by the kidneys is cleared by metabolism). The various route or organ clearances are additive, i.e.

$$CL_{renal} + CL_{extrarenal} = CL_{total}$$

Determination of clearance

In human pharmacokinetic studies, direct determination of whole body (systemic or plasma) clearance by the physiological approach, requiring, as it does, organ blood flow measurements and arterial and venous drug concentration determinations, is rarely possible. Whole body clearance is usually measured indirectly, using the relationship (see Chapter 3):

$$CL = \frac{DOSE}{AUC}$$

or

$$CL = k.V$$

The first of these relationships is model independent, and generally yields a constant value over the plasma or blood concentration range studied. However, for drugs that exhibit saturable or dose-dependent elimination, such clearance values will vary depending on drug concentration.

Determination of renal clearance (CL_R) is discussed in Chapter 2. It may be measured directly as the ratio of the concentration of drug in urine multiplied by the urine flow rate, to the concentration of drug in plasma at the mid-point of the urine collection interval. Alternatively, renal clearance may be calculated indirectly using the equation:

$$CL_R = fe(\infty).CL$$

where $fe(\infty)$ = the fraction of the drug dose excreted unchanged in urine.

For the great majority of drugs the difference between plasma clearance

(CL) and the renal clearance (CL_R) of unchanged drug represents a reasonable measure of the hepatic or metabolic clearance of the drug (since clearance values are additive):

$$CL_H = CL - CL_R$$

It should be noted that if a drug is given by other than the intravenous route there can be no certainty that the whole dose given enters the general circulation during the period of study. For orally administered drugs the degree to which the clearance value (CL_{oral}) exceeds the plasma clearance after intravenous administration ($CL_{i.v.}$) provides a measure of the extent to which the orally administered drug fails to be absorbed and/or is metabolized presystemically (in the gut wall and liver) before entering the general circulation.

Implications of clearance values

Interpretation of clearance values requires knowledge of whether a drug is eliminated chiefly by metabolism, or by excretion unchanged, as mentioned earlier. In the case of elimination predominantly by excretion unchanged, if the route of excretion is renal (as it nearly always is) renal clearance will approximate to whole body clearance. If urine is collected for a long enough time, the great majority of the dose given will be measurable as unchanged drug in that urine.

Drugs cleared by renal excretion unchanged – A substance cleared from blood plasma into urine solely by glomerular filtration (e.g. inulin) has a renal clearance of some 120 ml/min, i.e. approximately 7 l/h or $0.1\ l\ kg^{-1}\ h^{-1}$ (remembering that it is only drug not bound to plasma proteins that will be filtered into urine, so that the unbound drug concentration in plasma should be used for the clearance calculation). If the substance also undergoes net tubular resorption the clearance value will be less than this; if it undergoes active net tubular secretion into urine the clearance value will be higher and may reach a maximum corresponding to the value of renal plasma flow, around 560 ml/min (i.e. 34 l/h or about $0.5\ l\ kg^{-1}\ h^{-1}$). To obtain the most reliable information from renal clearance measurements in practice it may be desirable to produce a diuresis (by forced water drinking) at the time of the studies, and to measure clearance more than once, at different urine flow rates. This precaution reduces the risk that renal tubular secretion of a drug may happen to cancel out the effects of passive tubular resorption at the one urine flow rate studied, and thus to produce a clearance value which happens to be similar to the expected glomerular filtration rate, a finding which would suggest that the kidney excreted the drug by glomerular filtration alone. If renal clearance of drug in plasma water proves close to $0.1\ l\ kg^{-1}\ h^{-1}$ at a number of different rates of urine flow it is reasonable to infer that the drug is excreted purely by glomerular filtration. If the value is lower it may be inferred that the drug also undergoes passive tubular reabsorption (in which case clearance will rise with increased urine flow, though it will not exceed glomerular filtration rate). If clearance of drug in plasma water exceeds glomerular filtration rate at any rate of urine flow, it may be inferred that the drug undergoes active tubular secretion, whether or not it also undergoes passive tubular resorption. In these circumstances clearance values could be as high as $0.5 \, \text{l kg}^{-1} \, \text{h}^{-1}$ of whole plasma (or in theory even higher, if clearance is calculated on the basis of plasma water drug concentration, since tubular secretion may possibly be rapid enough to clear some drug that dissociates from plasma protein binding sites during passage of plasma along the renal tubule after the drug molecules in plasma water are all cleared).

The above comments apply to the situation when renal clearance is measured directly. However, conclusions in the same general direction can be drawn if whole plasma clearance is measured, and it is also known that the drug is eliminated unchanged and very largely or entirely by renal mechanisms.

Knowledge of how the kidney handles a drug may be useful to the clinician. Glomerular function diminishes with age, so that for drugs whose clearances are predominantly renal, the dose will often need to be reduced as the patient ages to lessen the risk of drug toxicity. If (relatively) selective tubular disease (e.g. crush syndrome) occurs, drugs excreted by active tubular secretion may accumulate more than those excreted purely by glomerular filtration. In diuresis, clearance will increase for drugs which undergo significant amounts of tubular resorption; this could lead to the need for increased doses to maintain biological effects if diuretic therapy is employed on a long-term basis. When peritoneal dialysis or haemodialysis is used in cases of severe renal insufficiency the non-protein-bound drug in plasma may be removed from the body, as it is in physiological circumstances by glomerular filtration. However, once removed by dialysis, the drug is lost to the body as there is no possibility of its subsequent reabsorption as might occur while the drug in urine passes down the renal tubules.

In the case of renal glomerular functional impairment, as in renal failure and in the elderly, attempts have been made to derive mathematical relationships which permit the estimation of an appropriate drug dose. One such method, described by Wagner (1975), depends on the fact that, in a given patient, a drug's elimination rate constant (k) is related to the creatinine clearance. The overall elimination rate constant (k) equals the sum of the rate constants for elimination by metabolism (k_m) and by renal excretion unchanged (k_r), i.e.

$$k = k_m + k_r$$

but

$$k_r = \frac{\text{CL}_{\text{drug,}}}{V} \quad \text{and if} \quad R = \frac{\text{CL}_{\text{drug}}}{\text{CL}_{\text{creatinine}}}$$

therefore

$$k = k_m + \frac{R \cdot CL_{creatinine}}{V}$$

The patient's creatinine clearance can be measured, or if only the serum creatinine is known, approximated from the relationships:

$$\text{for males } CL_{creatinine} \text{ (ml/min)} = \frac{(140\text{-age}) \times (\text{body weight})}{72 \text{ x serum creatinine concentration}}$$

$$\text{and for females } CL_{creatinine} \text{ (ml/min)} = \frac{(140\text{-age}) \times (\text{body weight})}{85 \text{ x serum creatinine concentration}}$$

The drug dose required is the normal dose multiplied by the ratio of k for the patient and for normal subjects.

$$\text{i.e. Dose required } = \text{ Normal dose } \times \frac{k(\text{patient})}{k(\text{normal})}$$

For most drugs $k(\text{normal})$ is known, and for certain drugs values of k_m and R/V are available for persons in renal failure. For the latter drugs substitution of the appropriate values in the above equations will permit calculation of expected dose. For drugs for which such k_m and R/V values are not known an approximate guide is still available in that the necessity of dose adjustment only arises when k_m is small in relation to the total elimination rate constant (k), i.e. drugs cleared mainly by renal excretion unchanged. For such drugs the $k(\text{patient})/k(\text{normal})$ ratio that determines dosage is approximated by the ratio:

$$\frac{\dfrac{R}{V} \cdot CL_{creatinine \text{ (patient)}}}{\dfrac{R}{V} \cdot CL_{creatinine \text{ (normal)}}} = \frac{k(\text{patient})}{k(\text{normal})}$$

Therefore, assuming V does not change in renal disease (this may not be so) the ratio of the patient's creatinine clearance to the well-known normal value of this parameter may provide a clinically useful guide to initial prescription of an appropriate drug dosage in persons with renal insufficiency.

Drugs cleared by excretion unchanged through non-renal mechanisms – Such situations are rarely studied in practice, except for gaseous anaesthetics in relation to the lungs. The same type of consideration would apply as for renally-cleared drugs, individual situations being interpreted in terms of the relevant physiology.

Drugs cleared by metabolism – Most drug metabolism is thought to occur in the liver, though metabolism may also occur in the gut wall, in the bloodstream (particularly hydrolysis of esters) and in other organs, e.g. the lungs and skin. For drugs which are eliminated almost entirely by metabolism, clearance values after intravenous dosage can approach the expected value of hepatic blood flow (96 l/h, or 1.4 l kg^{-1} h^{-1}). For certain drugs the capacity of hepatocytes to extract drug from blood and metabolize it is so great that, during a single passage of blood through the liver, all drug molecules in plasma water, bound to plasma protein and contained in the circulating cellular elements, may be extracted into hepatocytes and there metabolized. For such drugs, hepatic blood flow limits the amount of drug cleared and, therefore sets the limit to the value of clearance. For other drugs ('capacity-limited' drugs) clearance may be an order of magnitude, or more, lower than for the 'flow-limited' drugs. Hepatic metabolic capability limits the clearance of such capacity-limited drugs, rather than hepatic blood flow. The 'flow-limited' drugs include many of the narcotics (morphine, pethidine, but not methadone), many of the phenothiazines and tricyclic antidepressants, lignocaine, glyceryl trinitrate, endogenous oestrogen and testosterone, propranolol and ergotamine. In general, these are drugs which are recognized as being 'unreliable' if given by mouth, or having to be given in very much higher oral than parenteral doses to achieve a desired effect.

Hepatocyte disease, if not too severe, might not be expected to have any major effect on the clearance of 'flow-limited' drugs or on their dosage. However, liver cell disease would be likely to reduce the clearance of 'capacity-limited' drugs, and make dosage reduction necessary to avoid toxicity. Conversely, if liver blood flow was altered, as may occur in the intrahepatic blood shunting of cirrhosis, even though liver cell function remained relatively normal, clearance of 'flow-limited' drugs may be reduced more than clearance of 'capacity-limited' drugs. Dosage of 'flow-limited' drugs may then require appropriate modification to maintain a balance between therapeutic benefit and toxicity.

It is the 'flow-limited' drugs which are likely to undergo presystemic elimination when given by mouth. As explained earlier, for such drugs oral clearance (CL_{oral}) exceeds intravenous clearance (CL_{iv}), and the value of oral clearance may also come to exceed the value of hepatic blood flow. The effective oral dosage of such drugs exceeds the intravenous (and parenteral) dose (as it also does for drugs which, when given orally, are incompletely absorbed). The value of the intravenous clearance provides some indication as to whether presystemic clearance or incomplete absorption is more likely to account for impaired entry of orally administered drug into the general circulation (impaired bioavailability). If intravenous clearance exceeds 0.2–0.3 l kg^{-1} h^{-1} for a drug which undergoes little renal excretion unchanged, it is likely that the drug will undergo significant presystemic clearance when taken by mouth, and so be incompletely bioavailable. Its oral dose will be somewhat larger than its parenteral dose.

(Apparent) volume of distribution (V)

The unit of clearance is volume per unit time. Clearance thus involves a volume element and a time element. Where exponential kinetics can provide a reasonably valid description of the elimination process the time element is determined by the rate constant k or β, and the volume element is the apparent volume of distribution of the drug, i.e. $CL = V \times k$ or $V \times \beta$.

If one thinks of the likely actual physical distribution of an intravenously administered drug in the body one can see that, in the first seconds after its administration, it will probably have an expanding volume of distribution as it is carried around the circulation and becomes mixed with the circulating blood. If the drug is so hydrophilic and of such molecular dimensions that it never leaves the vascular compartment, within a few minutes or less its volume of distribution will become that of plasma (approximately 0.05 l/kg). If, however, the drug can diffuse into extravascular water, once there has been time for mixing, the drug's actual volume of distribution will become that of extracellular water (approximately 0.15 l/kg) or, if it also enters cells, that of total body water (approximately 0.50 l/kg). While the drug is in the process of diffusing into and through the extravascular and intracellular compartments, the drug's actual volume of distribution will be less than the volume of the appropriate physical compartment (or compartments). Unfortunately, once the drug diffuses outside the vascular compartment its calculated apparent volume of distribution may not correspond with its actual physical volume of distribution. The reason for this possible non- correspondence lies in the fact that calculation of the apparent volume of distribution assumes that the drug exists at the same concentration as in plasma throughout its entire actual volume of distribution, and in reality this may not be the case. The extravascular drug, by virtue of binding to tissue molecules or because of its own lipophilicity, may be at a much higher concentration than the drug in whole plasma. In this case the value of apparent volume of distribution will exceed that of the physical space in which the drug is actually distributed.

Thus apparent volume of distribution is a parameter whose interpretation may involve the conceptual difficulty that its value may not correspond to the value of the real physical space through which the drug is distributed.

Calculation of V

There are several ways of calculating V, and they may not yield exactly the same numerical value for the parameter in the one subject. None derives the actual physical volume of the drug's distribution: instead, each derives a fictional quantity which purports to describe the real volume. The various methods of derivation of V are described in Chapter 3.

Implications of V values

When one considers the different ways in which V can be calculated, and recognizes that probably none determines the drug's real physical volume of distribution within the body, one might wonder how much credence to give to estimated values of the parameter.

V values around 0.05 l/kg after intravenous dosage provide reasonable evidence that a drug is actually distributed throughout vascular water only. V values around 0.15 l/kg make it likely that the drug's actual distribution corresponds to extracellular water. V values in the range 0.4–0.6 l/kg may indicate that a drug is distributed throughout total body water, but such values could also arise with distribution throughout extracellular water, but with the drug being more highly concentrated in the extravascular compartment than in plasma. Values of V greatly in excess of the volume of total body water (e.g. values of 10–20 l/kg) can arise if the drug is sufficiently concentrated in the extravascular compartment (in interstitial or intracellular fluid, or in both). Such values are, of course, logically absurd in terms of physical reality but they do suggest the distribution pattern mentioned above.

V values then do provide limited and sometimes ambiguous information about how a drug is distributed in the body. However, they are useful in another way. If one knows the plasma drug level one wishes to achieve in a patient, one can use the relationship

$$\text{Dose} = V/C(0)$$

to estimate the dose that will produce a plasma level close to the value of $C(0)$ initially. This can be done so long as the value of V for the drug in the population is known and if the value of V in the patient being treated is not expected to be too deviant from the population norm.

Data are available concerning reported changes in apparent volumes of distribution (V) in various physiological and diseased states. However, translation of these alterations into changes in physical volumes of part of the body, and vice versa, can be uncertain. Thus, while it would be logical to expect the physical volumes of distribution of many drugs to increase in states of oedema, there are often no experimental data showing that apparent volumes of distribution change in these circumstances. V values are usually determined by further manipulation of two parameters which can be measured individually with reasonable precision, i.e. CL and k (or β). The calculation of V involves the errors in calculating both CL and the rate constant. With these potential experimental errors in the calculated value of V, and the ambiguities in the interpretation of the parameter's value, it becomes difficult to know how to assess altered V values in relation to, for example, age and disease. For instance, the halflives of several benzodiazepines increase (i.e. k decreases) with the patient's age, but clearances (and dosage requirements) remain unaltered, because of compensatory increases in calculated V values. Superficially, this result could be interpreted as suggesting that the physical volume of the aged body in which the drug is distributed is increased. In real physical terms this is unlikely, indeed often absurd. In view of the magnitude in the V change, the altered V values may probably reflect increased mean drug concentrations in the extravascular compartment in the elderly. The clinician always needs to retain a critical awareness of the assumptions underlying the concept of apparent volume of distribution. He should place a heavy mental emphasis on the word 'apparent', and he should realize that the parameter is likely to be, for his purposes, the least meaningful pharmacokinetic one.

Intercompartmental rate constants (microscopic rate constants)

Multicompartment models of drug distribution involve the concept of drug molecule transport between compartments. Such transport is almost always by means of passive diffusion and hence is adequately described by exponential kinetics. The intercompartmental rate constants, specified as to direction of movement between compartments, can be computed iteratively using the formulae set down for the various pharmacokinetic models (see Chapter 3). These microscopic rate constants can be used to calculate the expected time courses of drug concentrations within the various compartments. However, these calculations have rarely been subjected to verification by experimental measurement. There is difficulty in determining the correspondence which may exist between postulated compartments into which drugs are distributed and the real structures of animal anatomy. Therefore, the intercompartmental (transfer) rate constants tend to appear as numbers which cannot easily be related to things which have an established physical reality. These rate constants tend to be quoted in tabulations of pharmacokinetic data derived in experimental studies, but they are often not discussed further, perhaps because they seem to confer precision on something which is too nebulous to be acceptable to the mind that is conscious of the realities of human and animal anatomy.

Michaelis–Menten parameters (V_{max} and K_m)

The elimination of some drugs appears to be more validly described by Michaelis–Menten than by linear (exponential) kinetics. The Michaelis–Menten equation, familiar to students of biochemistry, relates the velocity of an enzyme-catalysed reaction to the maximum possible velocity of that reaction (V_{max}), to the substrate concentration (S) and to the Michaelis constant (K_m). The latter constant is the substrate concentration at which the reaction velocity (V) reaches half the value of V_{max}. Thus

$$V = \frac{V_{max} \cdot S}{K_m + S}$$

If such thinking is applied to the active transport or metabolism of a drug, S and K_m would refer to drug concentration at the relevant site or sites (and plasma drug concentration provides a measure of this concentration) while V and V_{max} would refer to amount transported or cleared in unit time, V_{max} measuring the maximum capacity of the process. Thus K_m would be the plasma drug concentration at which 50% of the V_{max} is achieved. Drugs whose elimination follows Michaelis–Menten kinetics have no elimination rate constant, and therefore strictly speaking no halflife, though apparent halflives can be calculated which vary with the range of drug concentrations studied. Since the effects of V are to produce changes in drug concentration, for pharmacokinetic purpose the Michaelis–Menten equation can be expressed in concentration terms, thus:

$$- \frac{dC}{dt} = \frac{V_{max} \cdot C}{K_m + C}$$

where $-dC/dt$ = rate of change in drug concentration and C = drug concentration at the time being considered. Alternatively, the equation can be expressed in integrated form:

$$C(0) - C = V_{max} \cdot t - K_m \cdot \log C(0)/C$$

where $C(0)$ = the original drug concentration.

If K_m is much larger than C, the equation,

$$-dC/dt = \frac{V_{max} \cdot C}{K_m + C} \text{reduces to} -dC/dt = \frac{V_{max} \cdot C}{K_m}$$

which is the form of the equation for a linear (exponential) process, i.e.

$$-dC/dt = k \cdot C$$

As explained earlier, if C is sufficiently small relative to K_m a simple exponential process provides a good approximation to the Michaelis–Menten kinetics which should apply for all drugs eliminated to any significant extent by metabolism. This latter situation is often present in clinical pharmacokinetic work, and explains why linear (exponential) kinetics can often be used successfully in place of Michaelis–Menten kinetics to interpret the time course of drug concentrations encountered therapeutically. Unless it is known that a drug is eliminated purely, or very substantially, by passive processes there is always the risk that exponential kinetics will not provide as valid an interpretation of the data as Michaelis–Menten kinetics would. This danger increases when one is dealing with higher levels of drug concentration (when C becomes closer to K_m or exceeds K_m), particularly for drugs which are eliminated mainly by metabolism. How does one know when Michaelis–Menten rather than linear kinetics should be used, despite the greater computational difficulties that are then involved?

The simple answer would be to use Michaelis–Menten kinetics on all occasions, except when it is known that drug transport and drug elimination occur entirely by passive transfer processes. Unfortunately such a policy is not a practicable solution at the present time. The computational problems in calculating Michaelis–Menten parameters (see Chapter 4) particularly with multicompartment models, cause one to prefer exponential kinetics whenever they seem capable of providing a reasonable interpretation of the data. The practical answers to the question of when to use Michaelis–Menten kinetics are therefore:

(1) when it is already known that for the drug concentration range under study Michaelis–Menten kinetics provide a better description of the data than do exponential kinetics,

(2) when the plot of the concentration vs. time data on semilogarithmic paper shows deviations from linearity (of the pattern illustrated in Figure 5.2) at higher drug concentrations, and

(3) when the terminal elimination halflife tends to be longer in the same subject when a higher dose of the drug is studied, as compared with a lower dose. This, of course, is simply stating (2) in another way. However, it reflects the fact that, unless a wide range of drug concentrations can be studied, departures from linearity may be obscured by experimental error in determining plasma drug concentrations. Formal kinetic studies at two drug doses in the same subject are the surest way of demonstrating departures from linear kinetics.

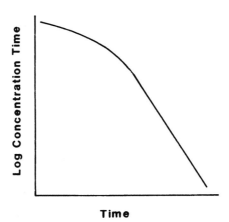

Figure 5.2 Semilogarithmic plot of the time course of declining plasma concentrations for a drug which is eliminated by a process that follows Michaelis–Menten kinetics

Calculation of Michaelis–Menten parameters

For the simplest case, that of elimination following Michaelis–Menten kinetics after intravenous administration of a drug, and when only the postdistributional phase decline in plasma drug concentrations is studied, (i.e. effectively a one-compartment model) the Michaelis–Menten equation is:

$$-dC/dt \ = \ \frac{V_{max} \cdot C}{K_m + C}$$

This equation can be written:

106

$$\frac{1}{(C(0)-C)/t} = \frac{1}{V_{max}} + \frac{K_m}{V_{max}} \cdot \frac{1}{C}$$

or

$$\frac{C}{(C(0)-C)/t} = \frac{K_m}{V_{max}} + \frac{1}{V_{max}} \cdot C$$

Both the equations immediately above are those for straight lines, of the

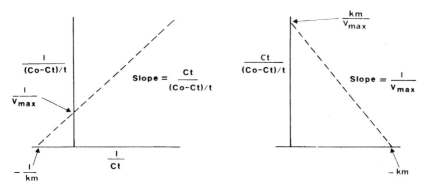

Figure 5.3 Graphical derivation of Michaelis–Menten parameters from plots of $1/(C(0)-C_t)$ against $1/C_t$ and of $C_t/(C(0)-C_t)t$ against C_t

form $y = a+bx$, and plots of the respective y vs. x values (Figure 5.3) permit graphical calculation of V_{max} and K_m.

The Michaelis–Menten based elimination equation can be solved iteratively with greater precision, after a numerical integration stage, using a computer. However, to obtain reliable values of V_{max} and K_m it is necessary to have plasma concentration vs. time data after two different doses of the drug given to the same individual (Metzler and Tong, 1981). With a single set of plasma concentration vs. time data, iterative fitting to the Michaelis–Menten equation in the form

$$-dC/dt = \frac{V_{max}.C}{K_m + C}$$

can become almost tantamount to fitting values of V_{max} and K_m to a V_{max}/K_m ratio, so that V_{max} and K_m can be varied almost in parallel over a very wide range of values to obtain slightly better fits to experimental data. Hence preposterous values of V_{max} and K_m can be obtained if the iteration is allowed to proceed without restraint. Yet any setting of limits to the parameters for the purpose of the iteration must be arbitrary. Other methods of determining Michaelis–Menten parameters have been described (Beal, 1982).

Relatively little has been published on the values of Michaelis–Menten elimination parameters of drugs in man. It seems generally accepted that, for practical purposes, very few of the drugs commonly used in human therapeutics deviate sufficiently from linear kinetics in the clinical situation for it to be desirable to use Michaelis–Menten kinetics to describe their plasma level behaviours. The two main exceptions are phenytoin and salicylate.

When the pharmacokinetic model is more complex than a one-compartment one with postdistributive elimination phase plasma concentration vs. time data only, e.g. when there is an absorption phase or a multicompartment distribution pattern, solution of the Michaelis–Menten parameters may be unsatisfactory even by computer methods. However, in these circumstances preliminary graphical estimation of V_{max} and K_m from the post-V_{max} distributional plasma level decline vs. time data can assist computation by providing reasonable parameter estimates to be entered into the iteration. With Michaelis–Menten elimination kinetics, should an attempt be made to calculate a clearance by dividing dose by AUC, one obtains a value that is not constant in the same individual at different plasma drug concentrations.

PARAMETERS RELATING TO DRUG ABSORPTION

The absorption halftime ($t_{\frac{1}{2},a}$) and the absorption rate constant (k_a) from which it is derived

The great majority of drugs are absorbed passively from their administration sites along concentration gradients. No active transport mechanism is involved. Passive transfer processes can be adequately described using exponential kinetics. In most circumstances drug absorption can be described adequately by a monoexponential process. The rate constant for this process is the absorption rate constant (k_a), and the corresponding halflife ($t_{\frac{1}{2},a}$) is calculated from the relationship:

$$t_{\frac{1}{2},a} = 0.693/k_a$$

The rate constant may be derived from the polyexponential equation of best fit to the plasma concentration vs. time data calculated as shown in Chapter 4, or may be determined less exactly by curve stripping (Chapter 4).

At times it may not be possible to describe drug absorption adequately in terms of simple monoexponential kinetics. Deviation from such kinetics may occur, for example, because

(1) there is a rate limiting step prior to the absorptive process, e.g. in the disintegration of a particular solid dosage form, or in the dissolution of its component molecules;

(2) absorption involves active transport, with its Michaelis–Menten type kinetics;

(3)   the drug under study may alter its own absorption, e.g. metoclopramide, which increases alimentary tract motility;

(4)   after initial absorption the drug may undergo an enterohepatic recirculation, so that a significant proportion of drug molecules enter the circulation on more than one occasion.

As mentioned in Chapter 4, the Wagner–Nelson method may still provide insight into the absorption process in these circumstances, so long as a one-compartment model is applicable. The absorption halftime and absorption rate constant may be valid for the particular set of circumstances in which they have been measured. However, particularly for orally administered drugs, the rate constants in the one individual may vary very considerably from occasion to occasion, depending on factors such as changing alimentary tract motility and the effects of food. Therefore, in practice the absorption parameters are not often very useful in guiding therapy. The values of these absorption parameters are not usually cited in tables of pharmacokinetic parameters of various drugs.

The absorption lag time (t_{lag})

There may be delay from the time a drug is administered to when it first appears in the blood. This delay represents the time for the drug to reach its absorption site from its administration site (if the two are different, as when a drug given by mouth is absorbed from the small intestine), plus any time occupied in actually entering the body and gaining entry to the bloodstream. Lag time can be determined graphically, or by computing (iteratively) the time when the plasma level value first leaves the baseline and then continues to rise with time.

Like the absorption rate constant and the absorption halftime, the lag time is likely to vary considerably from dose to dose in the one person. This variation results from the lag time depending both on pharmaceutical factors and on the vagaries of alimentary tract motility. The parameter may be valid in the circumstances in which it is measured, but these circumstances are often not readily reproducible, nor are the parameter values more generally applicable.

The t_{max} (time to achieve maximum concentration)

In thinking of the time course of the action of a given dose of a drug, it is clearly useful to know when the maximum effect of that dose is likely to occur. The time of maximum action will often coincide with the time of peak plasma drug concentration (the t_{max}). However, there may be delay in drug distribution to receptor sites or in receptor occupancy by drug molecules being transduced into a clinically apparent action of the drug. If so the time of maximum effect may be later than the t_{max}. Maximum effect may precede the t_{max} if the drug dose saturates all available receptors before the t_{max} is attained.

The t_{max} represents the moment when drug concentration in the body becomes high enough for elimination to equal absorption. Prior to this time absorption rate has exceeded elimination rate; after the t_{max} elimination will predominate. The t_{max} is not purely a function of absorption rate. If two drugs have identical absorption rates, but one drug is more slowly eliminated than the other, the drug with the slower elimination will have the later t_{max} (Figure 5.4).

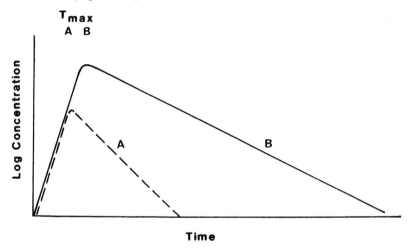

Figure 5.4 t_{max} occurs later for B than for A, despite identical absorption rates

The value of t_{max} is often read from the plasma level vs. time curve by interpolation. Sometimes the time of the highest measured plasma drug concentration is taken as the t_{max}, without interpolation. If linear absorption and elimination kinetics apply t_{max} can be calculated from the following formula for a one-compartment model.

$$t_{max} = \frac{1}{k_a - k} \cdot \log k_a/k$$

When the drug's kinetics are non-linear, it should be possible to calculate t_{max} iteratively from the equation of best fit to the plasma level vs. time data.

Because of variation in absorption rates from one person to the next, and within the one individual from time to time (with alteration in factors such as alimentary tract motility and local blood flow at the absorption site), t_{max} is a parameter which may have a rather wide range of values in the population. However, the t_{max} provides some guidance to time of expected maximum effect of a given drug dose.

Bioavailability (F)

The term 'bioavailability' refers to the rate and extent of a drug's appearance in the systemic (general) circulation, whence it becomes 'available' to the tissues of the body generally. Bioavailability is usually concerned mainly with the extent of drug entry to the general circulation. Rate of entry is important only when rapidity of action is a major concern. However, if rate of entry is slow enough the drug may not remain at its sites of entry for long enough for complete absorption to occur. The absorption rate constant is a commonly used measure of the entry rate aspect of bioavailability. For a drug given by mouth, with an alimentary tract transit time of, say, 24 h, an absorption rate constant below $0.087 \ h^{-1}$ (i.e. an absorption halftime of more than 8 h) would imply that one eighth of the dose given would not have time to be absorbed before the drug had been passed from the body. However, 8 h would be an unusually slow absorption halftime except for a slow-release or delayed-release preparation.

If a drug is injected directly into the systemic circulation it is immediately and completely bioavailable. As explained earlier, $AUC_{0 \to \infty}$ is a function of the drug dose entering the systemic circulation, and of the absorption, distribution and elimination parameters of the drug in a given individual. The same individual on one occasion may be given the drug in question by intravenous injection, and on another occasion by some other route e.g. by mouth. If there is no reason to suspect that his absorption, distribution and elimination parameters vary between the two studies (and these parameters can be determined experimentally from the same data used to calculate $AUC_{0 \to \infty}$), the ratio

$$\frac{AUC_{0 \to \infty} \cdot DOSE_{IV}}{AUC_{0 \to \infty (IV)} \cdot DOSE}$$

provides a measure of the bioavailability of the drug from the route of administration being studied. If the AUC after intravenous administration is used as the basis of comparison, the ratio refers to the so-called 'absolute' bioavailability. Where the drug is not given intravenously, and AUC comparisons are made between the drug given by two different routes, or in two different preparations by the same route, the ratio refers to the 'relative' bioavailability.

In bioavailability work it is necessary to show that the drug elimination rate constant remains the same when the drug is given by different routes, or in different preparations. The apparent elimination rate constant may change if the drug does not follow linear kinetics and if the two preparations studied deliver different quantities of drug into the general circulation. In this circumstance, if elimination involves a Michaelis–Menten kinetic stage (perhaps plus an exponential one) bioavailibility may be measured by calculating the values of V_{max}, K_m and k from the intravenous data, and then by determining the bioavailibility (F) from the relation defined by Martis and Levy (1973).

Incomplete bioavailability may arise because of (1) incomplete absorption and/or (2) metabolic destruction of part of the drug dose before it reaches the systemic circulation. Incomplete absorption can result from a drug preparation which releases its active substance too slowly, from a drug which is itself too insoluble, or from disease which affects the absorptive process. The first and second of these factors can often be remedied by better pharmaceutical preparations. Presystemic metabolism of drugs occurs in relation to oral administration and takes place in the alimentary tract wall and the liver. The process is referred to as presystemic elimination, or the 'first-pass' effect. It is a consequence of the body's interaction with the drug, and cannot be altered by changes in pharmaceutical preparation. It has also been discussed in relation to the concept of clearance (see above), where it was pointed out that drugs which have incomplete oral bioavailabilities due to presystemic elimination generally have high intravenous clearance values, and even higher oral clearance values. If the intravenous clearance is relatively low, e.g. below 0.2 l kg^{-1} h^{-1}, any incomplete bioavailability is likely to be due to poor drug absorption.

When drugs are incompletely bioavailable,

(1)   their effective oral doses are higher than their parenteral doses,
(2)   if the incomplete bioavailability is due to poor absorption, the drugs are also often inconsistently bioavailable. The amount absorbed after oral administration sometimes varies considerably with the vagaries of alimentary motility. Such drugs and drug preparations tend to yield variable degrees of pharmacological response from time to time and are generally undesirable in therapeutics.

Recommendations for the technical aspects of carrying out efficient bioavailability studies have been published (WHO report, 1974). In general such studies should employ assays of sufficient sensitivity and specificity, plasma concentration vs. time curves should be followed for at least three elimination halflives of the drug, and the same subjects should be crossed-over between the various drug preparations under test, with consecutive studies being carried out at a long enough interval for one drug dose not to interact with the next.

Contemporary drug regulatory authorities often require that a drug preparation has its bioavailability determined before marketing is permitted. As a result drug preparations introduced in recent times should have optimal bioavailabilities, but older preparations may not. If alternative brands of these older preparations come to be marketed, and prove more bioavailable than their predecessors, dosages of the newer preparation will need to be lower than dosages of the earlier preparation to avoid causing overdosage manifestations.

If incomplete bioavailability is due to presystemic elimination the occurrence of liver disease may increase the bioavailability of the drug, so that its dose may need to be reduced. (This, of course, is equivalent to saying that the metabolic clearance of the drug will fall.) If incomplete bioavailability is due to poor absorption of a drug, any disease process which increases alimentary tract motility may further decrease the bioavailability and therefore increase the dosage requirement.

References

Arnold, K. and Gerber, N. (1970). *Clin. Pharmacol. Ther.*, **11**, 121–34

Beal, S.L. (1982). *J. Pharmacokin. Biopharm.*, **10**, 109–19

Martis, L. and Levy, R.H. (1973). *J. Pharmacokin. Biopharm.*, **1**, 283–94

Metzler, C.M. and Tong, D.D.M. (1981). *J. Pharm. Sci.*, **70**, 733–37

Wagner, J. G. (1975). *Fundamentals of Clinical Pharmacokinetics*. (Hamilton: Drug Intelligence Publications)

WHO (1974). Bioavailability of drugs: principles and problems. *WHO Tech. Rep. Ser.*, *536*, 1–17

Appendix

Tutorial exercise – Apple II Microcomputer programs

If this tutorial is followed and the programs are all on a single floppy disk then the reader will be able to:

(1) enter data from Table 4.1,
(2) fit the data with a one-compartment i.v. bolus model,
(3) output calculated values to a disk file,
(4) produce a graph of the observed and calculated data.

All USER input is underlined.

Type RUN HELLO or enter PR#6
Choose 4 for the DATA.EDITOR – After this program has loaded – Enter <ctrl F> – Hold the ctrl and F keys down together Enter 2 <cr> for 2 fields (time and concentration) – press 2 then RETURN
Enter Time <cr>, enter Concentration <cr>
Enter 1 <cr> 22.3 <cr> 2 <cr> 17 <cr> 4 <cr> 14 <cr> 6 <cr> 10.3 <cr> 9 <cr> 6.9 <cr> 12<cr> 3.4 <cr> – this is the data from Table 4.1
Enter <ctrl P> and choose 2 screen to review the data
Press <cr>, enter <ctrl S> to save the data – Enter TABLE 4.1 <cr> <cr> <cr>
Press <ctrl C> <cr> to exit back to HELLO program
Choose 2 for to run the MULTI program – After this program has loaded – Enter 1 <cr> for DAMPING GAUSS–NEWTON METHOD
Enter TABLE 4.1 G–N <cr> for title
Enter Y <cr> for print out, enter 1 <cr> for the one-compartment i.v. bolus model, and enter 0 <cr> for equal weighting
Enter TABLE 4.1 <cr> and enter 0 1 and Y to confirm
Enter 0.001 <cr> for DT
Enter 0.16 <cr> 3.87 <cr> 100 <cr>
Once the print out is complete
Choose 4 <cr> and enter Y
The calculated data should now be stored as TABLE(110).CAL

Enter –1 <cr> to return to the HELLO program
Choose 3 for GRAPH.IT
After this program is loaded
Enter 12 <cr> for the x-axis, 0 <cr> for a linear plot, and 25 <cr> for the y-axis
Enter TABLE 4.1 <cr> to enter the experimental data and 0 1 Y <cr> to confirm the entry
After the plot press <cr> 1
Press <cr> for a CATALOG of the disk in drive 1
Enter TABLE(110).CAL <cr> to enter the calculated data and 0 1 Y<cr> to confirm the entry
After the plot press <cr> 3
Enter Table 4.1 G–N Equal Weighting <cr> to give a title for the plot
After the printout press 4 <cr> to return to the HELLO program and press 1 to exit

HELLO Program listing

```
10 TEXT : HOME
20 VTAB 4: PRINT "1) QUIT 2) MULTI": VTAB 6: PRINT "3)
        GRAPH.IT 4) DATA.EDITOR ";: GET T$: PRINT T$
30 IF T$ = "1" THEN TEXT : HOME : END
40 IF T$ = "2" THEN PRINT CHR$ (4);"RUN MULTI.PGM"
50 IF T$ = "3" THEN PRINT CHR$ (4);"RUN GRAPH.IT"
60 IF T$ = "4" THEN PRINT CHR$ (4);"RUN DATA.EDITOR"
70 GOTO 10
```

DATA.EDITOR Program Listing

```
1  REM  DATA.EDITOR
2  REM (C) 1985 D.W.A. BOURNE
3  REM 26 APRIL 85
10 TEXT : HOME : VTAB 2:T$ = "DATA EDITOR": GOSUB 900
12 VTAB 10:T$ = "DAVID W.A. BOURNE": GOSUB 900
14 VTAB 12:T$ = "DEPARTMENT OF PHARMACY": GOSUB 900
16 VTAB 14:T$ = "UNIVERSITY OF QUEENSLAND": GOSUB 900
18 FOR I = 1 TO 200: NEXT
20 MR = 199:MC = 19:MF = MC: REM MR MAXIMUM ROWS, MC
        NUMBER OF COLUMNS, MF MAXIMUM NUMBER OF
        COLUMNS(FIELDS)
22 CR = 0:CC = 0: REM CR CURRENT ROW, CC CURRENT
        COLUMN
24 FI$ = ""
30 DIM WD$(MR + 1,MC + 1)
100 TEXT : HOME : VTAB 2:T$ = "DATA EDITOR": GOSUB 900
130 POKE 34,3
140 POKE 35,20
```

```
150 VTAB 22: PRINT "PRESS '?' FOR HELP"
190 VTAB 4
200 REM START OF DATA ENTRY
210 GOSUB 800
220 HTAB (26): PRINT A$;: GET T$
225 IF T$ > CHR$ (26) THEN 280
230 IF T$ = CHR$ (13) THEN T$ = CHR$ (21)
235 IF T$ = CHR$ (08) THEN GOSUB 700:CC = CC - 1: PRINT :
        GOTO 200
240 IF T$ = CHR$ (21) THEN GOSUB 700:CC = CC + 1: PRINT :
        GOTO 200
245 IF T$ = CHR$ (10) THEN GOSUB 700:CR = CR + 1: PRINT :
        GOTO 200
250 IF T$ = CHR$ (11) THEN GOSUB 700:CR = CR - 1: PRINT :
        GOTO 200
265 IF T$ = CHR$ (4) AND A$ < > "" THEN A$ = MID$ (A$,1,
        LEN (A$) - 1): GOTO 200
270 IF T$ = CHR$ (19) THEN GOTO 1000: REM SAVE DATA LIST
271 IF T$ = CHR$ (16) THEN GOTO 3000: REM PRINT DATA LIST
272 IF T$ = CHR$ (3) THEN GOTO 4000: REM END
273 IF T$ = CHR$ (6) THEN GOTO 6000: REM DEFINE NUMBER
        OF FIELDS
274 IF T$ = CHR$ (20) THEN 7000: REM DATA
        TRANSFORMATION SECTION
275 IF T$ = CHR$ (12) THEN 2000: REM LOAD DATA LIST
277 IF T$ = CHR$ (14) THEN WD$(CR,CC) = "":A$ = "": GOSUB
        800: GOTO 200: REM ZERO ENTRY
280 IF T$ = "?" THEN 5000: REM HELP DISPLAY
300 A$ = A$ + T$: GOTO 220
600 REM S/R TO FIND NUMBER OF ROWS, RC
610 RC = 1
620 IF LEN (WD$(RC,0)) < > 0 THEN RC = RC + 1: GOTO 620
630 RC = RC - 1
640    RETURN
700 REM END OF ITEM
710 IF LEN (A$) = 0 THEN 730: REM NO CHANGE
720 WD$(CR,CC) = A$:A$ = ""
730    RETURN
800 REM S/R TO DISPLAY CURRENT WORD
802 IF CR > MR THEN CR = 0
804 IF CR < 0 THEN CR = MR
806 IF CC > MC THEN CC = 0:CR = CR + 1: GOTO 800
808 IF CC < 0 THEN CC = MC:CR = CR - 1: GOTO 800
810      HTAB      1:      PRINT      "          ";:
        HTAB 1: REM 38 SPACES
820 PRINT "ITEM ";: INVERSE : PRINT STR$ (CR);: NORMAL :
        HTAB 10: PRINT WD$(0,CC);: HTAB 26: PRINT
        WD$(CR,CC);
```

```
860    RETURN
900 REM CENTRE TEXT S/R
910 T = LEN (T$)
920 HTAB (40 – T) / 2: PRINT T$
930    RETURN
1000 REM SAVE DATA LIST SECTION
1010 TEXT : POKE 34,10: HOME
1020 VTAB 11:T$ = "SAVE DATA TO DISK": INVERSE : GOSUB
       900
1030 VTAB 13:T$ = "ENTER FILE NAME TO SAVE": GOSUB 900
1040 VTAB 14:T$ = "RETURN TO RE-EDIT": GOSUB 900:
       NORMAL
1042    PRINT
1044 ONERR GOTO 1400
1045 IF LEN (FI$) > 0 THEN T$ = "PRESS RETURN TO USE " +
       FI$: GOSUB 900
1050 PRINT : HTAB 15: INPUT T$
1055 IF LEN (T$) = 0 AND LEN (FI$) > 0 THEN 1090
1060 IF LEN (T$) = 0 THEN 100
1070 FI$ = T$
1090 RC = 0: REM ROW COUNT
1110 VTAB 19:T$ = "INSERT DATA DISK": GOSUB 900
1120 VTAB 20:T$ = " PRESS RETURN": HTAB ((40 – LEN (T$)) /
       2): PRINT T$;: NORMAL
1130 GET T$: PRINT T$
1140 GOSUB 600
1180 PRINT "PRESS RETURN TO CONTINUE, ANY OTHER KEY
       TO EXIT ";: GET T$: PRINT T$: IF T$ = CHR$ (13) THEN
       GOTO 1200
1190 CR = 1:CC = 0: GOTO 100
1200 PRINT CHR$ (4);"OPEN ";FI$
1210 PRINT CHR$ (4);"WRITE ";FI$
1215 PRINT RC: PRINT MC: PRINT FI$: REM NUMBER OF ROWS,
       NUMBER OF COLUMNS(+1) AND FILE NAME
1220 FOR I = 0 TO RC
1230 FOR J = 0 TO MC: PRINT WD$(I,J): NEXT J:
1240 NEXT I
1340 PRINT CHR$ (4);"CLOSE ";FI$
1350 POKE 216,0: RUN
1360    END
1400 REM SAVE I/O ERROR SECTION
1410 TEXT : HOME
1420 VTAB 10: PRINT "ERROR WHILE SAVING DATA"
1430 PRINT : PRINT "POSSIBLE CAUSES INCLUDE NO ROOM ON
       DATA  DISK"
1490 PRINT : PRINT "PRESS RETURN TO TRY AGAIN ";: INPUT
       T$: GOTO 1000
2000 REM LOAD DATA SECTION
```

```
2010 TEXT : POKE 34,10: HOME : VTAB 11
2020 T$ = "LOAD DATA TO DISK": INVERSE : GOSUB 900
2030 PRINT :T$ = "ENTER FILE NAME:- ": GOSUB 900
2040 T$ = "PRESS RETURN TO CATALOG": GOSUB 900: NORMAL
2050 PRINT : HTAB 15: INPUT T$
2060 IF LEN (T$) = 0 THEN PRINT CHR$ (4);"CATALOG": GOTO
     2020
2070 FI$ = T$
2100   FLASH
2110 PRINT :T$ = "INSERT DATA DISK": GOSUB 900
2120 T$ = " PRESS RETURN": GOSUB 900: NORMAL
2130 HTAB 19: GET T$: PRINT T$
2200 PRINT CHR$ (4);"OPEN ";FI$
2210 PRINT CHR$ (4);"READ ";FI$
2220 INPUT  RC,MC,T$
2225 FOR I = 0 TO RC
2230 FOR J = 0 TO MC: INPUT WD$(I,J): NEXT J
2240 NEXT I
2400 PRINT CHR$ (4);"CLOSE "FI$
2410 GOTO 100
3000 REM PRINT DATA LIST
3010 TEXT : HOME
3020 VTAB 10:T$ = "REVIEW DATA ON SCREEN OR PRINTER":
     GOSUB 900
3030 VTAB 15: PRINT "1) PRINTER"
3040 PRINT "2) SCREEN"
3050 PRINT "3) RETURN"
3060 PRINT : INPUT "ENTER CHOICE ";T$
3070 IF T$ = "3" GOTO 100
3080 GOSUB 600
3090 IF T$ = "1" GOTO 3500
3100 IF T$ < > "2" GOTO 3000
3110 SPEED= 150
3120 FOR I = 0 TO RC
3130 PRINT : PRINT "DATA ";I; TAB( 10);"FIELD"; TAB(26);
     "VALUE": PRINT
3140 FOR J = 0 TO MC
3150 PRINT TAB( 10);WD$(0,J); TAB( 26);WD$(I,J)
3160 NEXT J
3165 T = PEEK ( - 16384) - 128: POKE - 16368,0: IF T > 0 THEN I
     = RC
3170 NEXT I
3180 SPEED= 255
3190 PRINT : PRINT "PRESS RETURN TO CONTINUE ";: INPUT
     T$
3200 GOTO 100
3500 REM  PRINTER  PATH
3510 PRINT : PRINT "SET-UP PRINTER AND PRESS RETURN";:
     INPUT  T$
```

```
3520 PRINT CHR$ (4);"PR#1"
3530 PRINT CHR$ (9);"132N": PRINT CHR$ (15)
3540 T = 24
3550 FOR J = 0 TO MC
3560 POKE 36,T: PRINT WD$(0,J);:T = T + 15
3570 IF T > 117 THEN T = T - 104: PRINT
3580 NEXT J: PRINT : PRINT
3590 FOR I = 1 TO RC
3600 T = 24: POKE 36,10: PRINT "DATA ";I;
3610 FOR J = 0 TO MC
3620 POKE 36,T: PRINT WD$(I,J);:T = T + 15
3630 IF T > 117 THEN T = T - 104: PRINT
3640 NEXT J: PRINT
3650 NEXT I: PRINT
3660 PRINT CHR$ (18): PRINT CHR$ (4);"PR#0"
3670 GOTO 100
4000  REM  END  ROUTINE
4010 TEXT : HOME
4020 VTAB 10:T$ = "PRESS RETURN TO FINISH": GOSUB 900
4030 VTAB 12:T$ = "ANY OTHER KEY TO CONTINUE": GOSUB
     900
4040 VTAB 14: HTAB 19: GET T$: PRINT T$
4050 IF T$ = CHR$ (13) THEN TEXT : HOME : PRINT CHR$
     (4);"RUN  HELLO,D1"
4060 TEXT : HOME : GOTO 100
5000  REM  HELP  DISPLAY
5010 PRINT : PRINT
5020 PRINT "CONTROL CHARACTERS ARE ENTERED BY
     HOLDING THE 'CTRL' KEY AND THE DESIGNATED
     LETTER DOWN TOGETHER. PRESS 'CTRL' AND 'C' TO
     ENTER '∧C'."
5030 PRINT : PRINT "USE 'RETURN' OR ARROWS TO ACCEPT
     DATA"
5035 PRINT "USE ARROWS TO MOVE IN THE DATA LIST"
5040  PRINT : PRINT "'∧D/∧N' TO DELETE CHARACTER/
     ENTRY"
5045 PRINT "'∧T/∧P' TO TRANSFORM/PRINT DATA"
5060 PRINT "'∧C' TO EXIT THE PROGRAM"
5065 PRINT "'∧F' TO DEFINE NUMBER OF FIELDS"
5070 PRINT "'∧S' OR '∧L' TO SAVE OR LOAD A DATA LIST"
5099 GOTO 200
6000 REM DEFINE THE NUMBER OF FIELDS
6010 HOME : VTAB 4
6020 PRINT "ENTER THE NUMBER OF FIELDS ";
6030 INPUT T$:MC = VAL (T$) - 1
6040 IF MC > MF THEN PRINT CHR$ (7): PRINT "THE MAXIMUM
     NUMBER OF FIELDS IS ";MF: GOTO 6000
6050 TEXT : HOME : GOTO 100
```

```
7000 REM DATA TRANSFORMATION SECTION
7010 TEXT : HOME
7020 VTAB 2:T$ = "DATA TRANSFORMATION": GOSUB 900
7030 PRINT : PRINT "NEW FIELD = "
7031 PRINT : PRINT "1) OLD FIELD + CONSTANT"
7032 PRINT "2) OLD FIELD x CONSTANT"
7033 PRINT "3) OLD FIELD(1) + OLD FIELD(2)"
7034 PRINT "4) OLD FIELD(1) - OLD FIELD(2)"
7035 PRINT "5) OLD FIELD(1) * OLD FIELD(2)"
7036 PRINT "6) OLD FIELD(1) / OLD FIELD(2)"
7037 PRINT "7) LOG(E) OLD FIELD(1)"
7038 PRINT "8) LOG(10) OLD FIELD(1)"
7039 PRINT "9) 1/OLD FIELD(1)"
7040 PRINT "10) SIN(OLD FIELD(1))"
7041 PRINT "11) OLD FIELD(1) ∧ CONSTANT"
7042 PRINT "12) EXP(OLD FIELD(1))"
7043 PRINT "13) ABS(OLD FIELD(1))"
7050 PRINT : INPUT "ENTER CHOICE ";T$:T = VAL (T$): IF T >
       13 OR T < 0 THEN 7000
7051 IF T = 0 THEN 100
7052 IF T > 13 THEN 7060: REM BY-PASS CHECK ON MAXIMUM
       COLUMNS
7053 MC = MC + 1: IF MC > MF THEN PRINT "ALREADY ";MF;"
       FIELDS": GOTO 7000
7055 PRINT : INPUT "ENTER FIELD DESCRIPTOR FOR NEW
       FIELD ";WD$(0,MC)
7060 ON T GOTO 7100,7100,7300,7300,7300,7300,7400,7400,
       7400,7400,7400,7400,7400,7500,7600,7700
7100 REM OLD FIELD +/* CONSTANT
7110 PRINT : FOR J = 0 TO MC - 1: PRINT J;") ";WD$(0,J): NEXT
7112 PRINT : INPUT "ENTER OLD FIELD NUMBER ";XI
7114 PRINT : INPUT "ENTER CONSTANT ";ZI
7116 GOSUB 600
7118 FOR I = 1 TO RC
7120 IF T = 1 THEN WD$(I,MC) = STR$ ( VAL (WD$(I,XI)) + ZI)
7121 IF T = 2 THEN WD$(I,MC) = STR$ ( VAL (WD$(I,XI)) * ZI)
7122  NEXT
7124  GOTO 100
7300 REM OLD FIELD +/* OLD FIELD
7302 PRINT : FOR J = 0 TO MC - 1: PRINT J;") ";WD$(0,J): NEXT
7304 PRINT : INPUT "ENTER OLD FIELD NUMBER(1) ";XI
7306 PRINT : INPUT "ENTER OLD FIELD NUMBER(2) ";ZI
7308 GOSUB 600
7310 FOR I = 1 TO RC
7312 IF T = 3 THEN WD$(I,MC) = STR$ ( VAL (WD$(I,XI)) + VAL
       (WD$(I,ZI))): GOTO 7318
7313 IF T = 4 THEN WD$(I,MC) = STR$ ( VAL (WD$(I,XI)) - VAL
       (WD$(I,ZI))): GOTO 7318
```

```
7314 IF T = 5 THEN WD$(I,MC) = STR$ ( VAL (WD$(I,XI)) * VAL
     (WD$(I,ZI))): GOTO 7318
7315 IF VAL (WD$(I,ZI)) = 0 THEN WD$(I,MC) = "* ERROR * /0":
     GOTO 7318
7316 IF T = 6 THEN WD$(I,MC) = STR$ ( VAL (WD$(I,XI)) / VAL
     (WD$(I,ZI)))
7318   NEXT
7319 GOTO 100
7400 REM OLD FIELD TRANSFORMED
7402 PRINT : FOR J = 0 TO MC – 1: PRINT J;") ";WD$(0,J): NEXT
7404 PRINT : INPUT "ENTER OLD FIELD NUMBER(1) ";XI
7408 IF T = 11 THEN PRINT : INPUT "ENTER CONSTANT ";ZI
7410 GOSUB 600
7420 FOR I = 1 TO RC
7422 ON T – 6 GOTO 7424,7424,7430,7432,7424,7434,7436
7424 IF VAL (WD$(I,XI)) < = 0 THEN WD$(I,MC) = "* ERROR*
     LOG(0)": GOTO 7498
7425 IF T = 7 THEN WD$(I,MC) = STR$ ( LOG ( VAL (WD$(I,XI)))):
     GOTO 7498
7426 IF T = 8 THEN WD$(I,MC) = STR$ ( LOG ( VAL (WD$(I,XI)))
     / LOG (10)): GOTO 7498
7427 IF T = 11 THEN WD$(I,MC) = STR$ ( VAL (WD$(I,XI)) ∧ ZI):
     GOTO 7498
7430 IF VAL (WD$(I,XI)) = 0 THEN WD$(I,MC) = "* ERROR* /0":
     GOTO 7498
7431 WD$(I,MC) = STR$ (1 / ( VAL (WD$(I,XI)))): GOTO 7498
7432 WD$(I,MC) = STR$ ( SIN ( VAL (WD$(I,XI)))): GOTO 7498
7434 WD$(I,MC) = STR$ ( EXP ( VAL (WD$(I,XI)))): GOTO 7498
7436 WD$(I,MC) = STR$ ( ABS ( VAL (WD$(I,XI)))): GOTO 7498
7498   NEXT
7499 GOTO 100
```

MULTI program listing

```
1 REM MULTI.PGM
2 REM 14 MAY 85
3 REM

      MULTI

      K.YAMAOKA,  Y.TANIGAWARA,
      T.NAKAGAWA,  AND  T.UNO
      J.PHARM.DYN., 4, 879–885 (1981)
4 REM MODIFIED BY D.W.A.BOURNE
```

122

5 REM

10 TEXT : HOME : VTAB 4: PRINT "* MULTI-LINES FITTING MARCH 29, 1981 *"

20 PRINT : PRINT "SELECT MODEL OR DEFINE EQUATIONS AT 1110, 1120, 1130, 1140 AND 1150": PRINT

30 PRINT "CP AND T ARE DEPENDENT AND INDEPENDENT VARIABLES, RESPECTIVELY"

35 PRINT "P(1), P(2), .. ARE THE PARAMETERS TO FIT"

36 PRINT : PRINT TAB(8);"GOTO 840 IF DIVERGED.":FP = 0

37 DIM ME$(3):ME$(0) = "GAUSS–NEWTON":ME$(1) = "DAMPING GAUSS–NEWTON

38 ME$(2) = "MARQUARDT":ME$(3) = "SIMPLEX"

40 PRINT : FOR I = 0 TO 3: PRINT "(";I;") ";ME$(I);" METHOD": NEXT

45 PRINT : INPUT "WHICH ALGORITHM DO YOU SELECT ";AL

49 PRINT : PRINT "–CONTINUE ONLY IF EQUATIONS ARE DEFINED–"

50 INPUT "TITLE? ";N$: INPUT "PRINT (Y/N)? ";P$

52 GOTO 11400

54 INPUT "NUMBER OF LINES ";LN: DIM NL(LN)

55 INPUT "NUMBER OF PARAMETERS ";M: INPUT "NUMBER OF CONSTANT";NC: INPUT "MODEL DESCRIPTION"; MD$

56 PRINT : INPUT "WEIGHT FOR DATA (0,1,2) ";IW

60 DIM A(M,M + 1),P(M),X(M,M),CN(NC)

62 GOSUB 9000

65 NL(0) = 0:BS = 0: FOR J = 1 TO LN:BS = BS + NL(J – 1): PRINT

70 PRINT "FOR LINE ";J: PRINT : PRINT "DATA #"; TAB(10);RD$(XI(J)); TAB(25);RD$(YI(J)): PRINT : FOR I = 1 TO NL(J): PRINT " ";I; TAB(12);TX(BS + I); TAB(27);CY(BS + I): NEXT I

75 NEXT J: IF AL = 3 THEN 3000

77 PC = 0.0001:CF = 100: IF FP = 0 THEN DIM CS(N,M):FP = 1

78 PRINT : INPUT "DT FOR JACOBIAN (0.1 to 0.0001) ";DT: PRINT

80 FOR I = 1 TO M: PRINT "INITIAL ";PL$(I);" = ";: INPUT A(I,0):P(I) = A(I,0): NEXT

90 IF NC > 0 THEN FOR I = 1 TO NC: PRINT "ENTER ";CN$(I);" = ";: INPUT CN(I): NEXT

100 GOSUB 4000:S1 = SS

140 PRINT "INITIAL SS = ";SS: FOR K = 1 TO 100: GOSUB 7000: GOSUB 7400: GOSUB 6000:JJ = 0

490 JJ = JJ + 1: IF JJ > 25 THEN 730

500 FOR I = 1 TO M:P(I) = A(I,0) + A(I,M + 1): NEXT : GOSUB 4000

510 DS = ABS (S1 – SS): IF AL < > 2 OR SS = 0 THEN 590

515 REM FLETCHER MODIFICATION

520 PW = 0: FOR I = 1 TO M:PW = PW + X(I,0) * A(I,M + 1) + CF * A(I,M + 1) * A(I,M + 1): NEXT

```
530 IF DS / PW > .75 THEN CF = CF / 2
540 IF DS / PW < .25 THEN CF = 5 * CF
590 IF DS < = PC * S1 THEN 730: REM CHECK OF CONVERGENCE
595  REM  DAMPING
600 IF AL = 1 AND SS > S1 THEN FOR I = 1 TO M:A(I,M + 1) =
    .5 * A(I,M + 1): NEXT : GOTO 490
630 FOR I = 1 TO M:A(I,0) = P(I): NEXT :S1 = SS: PRINT : PRINT
    "LOOP = ";K
640 IF AL = 1 THEN PRINT "DAMP = ";JJ
660 FOR I = 1 TO M: PRINT PL$(I);" = ";P(I): NEXT : PRINT "SS
    = ";SS:  NEXT
730 IF P$ = "y" OR P$ = "Y" THEN PRINT CHR$ (4);"PR#1":
    REM CHANGE TO PRINTER
731 PRINT : PRINT "* ";N$;" * BY ";ME$(AL);" METHOD": PRINT
    "MODEL  -  ";MD$:  PRINT  :  PRINT  "WEIGHT  =
    1/CP∧(";IW;")"
733 IF AL < > 3 AND N > M THEN GOSUB 8000
734 IF SS = 0 THEN PRINT "A.I.C. = –INFINITY": GOTO 740
735 PRINT "A.I.C. = ";N * LOG (SS) + 2 * M
740 IF AL = 3 THEN PRINT "ALPHA = ";AA;" BETA = ";BB;"
    AND GAMMA = ";CC: PRINT
742 IF AL < > 3 THEN PRINT "DT = ";DT
745 IF AL = 2 THEN PRINT "FACTOR = ";CF
747 IF NC > 0 THEN PRINT : PRINT "WITH:-": FOR I = 1 TO NC:
    PRINT CN$(I);" = ";CN(I): NEXT : PRINT
750 FOR I = 1 TO M: PRINT "FINAL ";PL$(I);" = ";P(I);
760 IF AL < > 3 AND X(I,0) > 0 AND N > M THEN PRINT "
    S.D. = "; SQR (X(I,0) * SS / (N – M));
810 PRINT : NEXT : PRINT : GOSUB 10000:BS = 0: FOR J = 1 TO
    LN:BS = BS + NL(J – 1)
820 PRINT : PRINT "FOR LINE ";J: PRINT : PRINT "DATA #";
    TAB( 10);RD$(XI(J)); TAB( 25);RD$(YI(J)); TAB(
    38);"(CALCULATED)": PRINT : FOR I = 1 TO NL(J):T =
    TX(BS + I): GOSUB 1000
830 PRINT " ";I; TAB( 12);T; TAB( 27);CP; TAB( 39);" (";CY(BS +
    I);")": NEXT I,J
832  GOSUB 11000
835 IF P$ = "y" OR P$ = "Y" THEN PRINT CHR$ (4);"PR#0":
    REM CHANGE TO CRT
840 PRINT : HOME : PRINT "MENU": PRINT : PRINT "–1) EXIT":
    PRINT " 0) REPEAT WITH GAUSS–NEWTON": PRINT " 1)
    REPEAT WITH DAMPING G–N": PRINT " 2) MAR-
    QUARDT": PRINT " 3) SIMPLEX": PRINT " 4) OUTPUT
    DATA FOR
    GRAPH.IT": PRINT " 5) NEW CALCULATION": PRINT :
    PRINT "ENTER CHOICE (–1,1,2,3,4,5)";
850 INPUT TA: IF TA < 0 THEN PRINT CHR$ (4);"RUN
    HELLO,D1"
```

124

```
855 IF TA = 5 THEN RUN
860 IF TA = 3 THEN AL = 3: GOTO 3000
870 IF TA = 4 THEN GOSUB 11200: GOTO 840
880 IF TA < > 0 AND TA < > 1 AND TA < > 2 THEN 840
890 IF AL < > 3 THEN AL = TA: GOTO 77
900 AL = TA:PC = 0.0001:CF = 100:DT = 0.0001: IF FP = 0 THEN
    DIM CS(N,M):FP = 1
910 FOR I = 1 TO M:A(I,0) = P(I): NEXT I: GOSUB 4000:S1 = SS:
    GOTO 140
1000 ON MD GOTO 1010,1020,1030,1040,1050,1060,1100
1010 CP = CN(1) * EXP ( - P(1) * T) / P(2): RETURN
1011 REM P(1) = KEL:P(2) = V:CN(1) = DOSE
1020 TINF = CN(1): IF T < TINF THEN TINF = T
1021 CP = CN(2) * (1 - EXP ( - P(1) * TINF)) * EXP ( - P(1) *
     (T - TINF)) / (P(1) * P(2)): RETURN
1022 REM P(1) = KEL:P(2) = V:CN(1) = INFUSION
     DURATION:CN(2) = INFUSION RATE
1030 CP = (CN(1) * P(2) / (P(3) * (P(2) - P(1)))) * ( EXP ( -
     P(1) * T) - EXP ( - P(2) * T)): RETURN
1031 REM P(1) = KEL:P(2) = KA:P(3) = V:CN(1) = DOSE
1040 CP = P(1) * EXP ( - P(2) * T) + P(3) * EXP ( - P(4) * T):
     RETURN
1041 REM P(1) = A:P(2) = ALPHA:P(3) = B:P(4) = BETA
1050   RETURN
1060   RETURN
1100 ON J GOTO 1110,1120,1130,1140,1150
1109 REM YOUR EQUATIONS
1110 REM DEFINE CP = F1(T,P(I)):RETURN
1120 REM DEFINE CP = F2(T,P(I)):RETURN
1130 REM DEFINE CP = F3(T,P(I)):RETURN
1140 REM DEFINE CP = F4(T,P(I)):RETURN
1150 REM DEFINE CP = F5(T,P(I)):RETURN
1999   REM JACOBIAN ************************
2000 FOR JS = 1 TO M:PT = P(JS):P(JS) = PT + DT: GOSUB 1000
2020 DD = CP:P(JS) = PT - DT: GOSUB 1000
2030 CS(BS + I,JS) = (DD - CP) / (2 * DT):P(JS) = PT: NEXT :
     RETURN
2999   REM SIMPLEX METHOD
3000 AA = 1:BB = .5:CC = 2:SG = 1E10:PC = .00001
3025 PRINT : FOR I = 1 TO M: PRINT "INITIAL ";PL$(I);" ";: INPUT
     A(I,1):   NEXT
3030 FOR J = 2 TO M + 1: FOR I = 1 TO M:A(I,J) = 2 * RND (1) *
     A(I,1) + .01 * ( RND (1) - .5): NEXT I,J
3040 FOR K = 1 TO M + 1: FOR I = 1 TO M:P(I) = A(I,K): NEXT :
     GOSUB 4000:A(0,K) = SS: NEXT
3070 PRINT : FOR I = 1 TO M + 1: PRINT "SS ";I;" = ";A(0,I):
     NEXT : GOTO 5000
3080 SR = 0:SL = 1E10: FOR J = 1 TO M + 1: IF SR < A(0,J) THEN
     JH = J:SR = A(0,J)
```

3090 IF SL > A(0,J) THEN JL = J:SL = A(0,J)
3100 NEXT :SR = 0: FOR J = 1 TO M + 1: IF J < > JH AND SR <
    A(0,J) THEN JS = J:SR = A(0,J)
3110 NEXT : FOR I = 1 TO M:X(0,I) = 0: FOR J = 1 TO M + 1: IF J
    < > JH THEN X(0,I) = X(0,I) + A(I,J)
3120 NEXT :X(0,I) = X(0,I) / M: NEXT : FOR I = 1 TO M:A(I,0) =
    (1 + AA) * X(0,I) – AA * A(I,JH)
3130 P(I) = A(I,0): NEXT : GOSUB 4000:SR = SS: IF SR < = A(0,JS)
    THEN 3300
3160 IF SR < A(0,JH) THEN FOR I = 1 TO M:A(I,JH) = A(I,0):
    NEXT :A(0,JH) = SR
3170 FOR I = 1 TO M:A(I,0) = BB * A(I,JH) + (1 – BB) * X(0,I)
3180 P(I) = A(I,0): NEXT : GOSUB 4000:SR = SS
3190 IF SR < A(0,JH) THEN FOR I = 1 TO M:A(I,JH) = A(I,0):
    NEXT :A(0,JH) = SR: GOTO 3070
3200 FOR K = 1 TO M + 1: FOR I = 1 TO M:A(I,K) = (A(I,K) +
    A(I,JL)) / 2:P(I) = A(I,K): NEXT
3210 GOSUB 4000:A(0,K) = SS: NEXT : GOTO 3070
3300 IF SR < A(0,JL) THEN 3500
3320 FOR I = 1 TO M:A(I,JH) = A(I,0): NEXT :A(0,JH) = SR: GOTO
    3070
3500 FOR I = 1 TO M:X(1,I) = CC * A(I,0) + (1 – CC) *
    X(0,I):P(I) = X(1,I): NEXT : GOSUB 4000:SL = SS
3510 IF SL < SR THEN FOR I = 1 TO M:A(I,JH) = X(1,I): NEXT
    :A(0,JH) = SL: GOTO 3070
3520 GOTO 3320
3999 REM CALCULATION OF SS
4000 SS = 0:BS = 0: FOR J = 1 TO LN:BS = BS + NL(J – 1): FOR I =
    1 TO NL(J):T = TX(BS + I)
4020 GOSUB 1000: IF CY(BS + I) < > 0 THEN SS = SS + (CY(BS +
    I) – CP) ∧ 2 / CY(BS + I) ∧ IW
4030 NEXT I,J: RETURN
4999 REM CHECK OF CONVERGENCE
5000 SR = 0: FOR I = 1 TO M + 1:SR = SR + A(0,I): NEXT
5030 IF ABS (SR – SG) > PC * SG THEN SG = SR: GOTO 3080
5040 FOR I = 1 TO M:P(I) = A(I,JL): NEXT :SS = A(0,JL): GOTO
    730
5999 REM GAUSS ELIMINATION WITH PIVOT
6000 IF NP = 1 THEN A(1,2) = A(1,2) / A(1,1): RETURN
6020 RM = ABS (A(1,1)): FOR IS = 1 TO NP: FOR JS = 1 TO NP
6050 IF RM < ABS (A(JS,IS)) THEN RM = ABS (A(JS,IS))
6060 NEXT JS,IS: FOR KS = 1 TO NP – 1:W = 0: FOR IS = KS TO
    NP
6100 IF ABS (A(IS,KS)) < W THEN 6130
6110 W = ABS (A(IS,KS)):JS = IS
6130 NEXT : IF JS = KS THEN 6200
6150 FOR IS = KS TO NP + 1:W = A(KS,IS):A(KS,IS) =
    A(JS,IS):A(JS,IS) = W: NEXT

6200 P = 1 / A(KS,KS): FOR JS = KS + 1 TO NP + 1:A(KS,JS) = A(KS,JS) * P:W = - A(KS,JS)

6250 IF W = 0 THEN 6290

6260 FOR IS = KS + 1 TO NP:A(IS,JS) = A(IS,JS) + A(IS,KS) * W: NEXT

6290 NEXT : NEXT :A(NP,NP + 1) = A(NP,NP + 1) / A(NP,NP): FOR IS = 2 TO NP

6350 LS = NP - IS + 1:W = - A(LS,NP + 1): FOR JS = LS + 1 TO NP

6400 W = W + A(LS,JS) * A(JS,NP + 1): NEXT :A(LS,NP + 1) = - W: NEXT : RETURN

6999 REM NORMAL EQUATION

7000 NL(0) = 0:BS = 0: FOR J = 1 TO LN:BS = BS + NL(J - 1): FOR I = 1 TO NL(J):T = TX(BS + I)

7300 GOSUB 1000:CS(BS + I,0) = CY(BS + I) - CP: GOSUB 2000

7310 NEXT I,J: FOR I = 1 TO M: FOR J = I TO M:A(I,J) = 0: FOR L = 1 TO N

7390 IF CY(L) < > 0 THEN A(I,J) = A(I,J) + CS(L,I) * CS(L,J) / CY(L) ∧ IW

7395 NEXT :A(J,I) = A(I,J): NEXT J,I: RETURN

7400 FOR I = 1 TO M:A(I,M + 1) = 0: FOR J = 1 TO N

7440 IF CY(J) < > 0 THEN A(I,M + 1) = A(I,M + 1) + CS(J,I) * CS(J,0) / CY(J) ∧ IW

7445 NEXT J,I:NP = M

7450 REM MARQUARDT MODIFICATION

7460 IF AL = 2 THEN FOR I = 1 TO M:A(I,I) = A(I,I) + CF:X(I,0) = A(I,M + 1): NEXT

7470 RETURN

7999 REM VARIANCE

8000 GOSUB 7000: FOR I = 1 TO M: FOR J = 1 TO M:X(I,J) = A(I,J): NEXT J,I

8010 FOR K = 1 TO M: FOR I = 1 TO M: FOR J = 1 TO M:A(I,J) = X(I,J): NEXT J,I: FOR I = 1 TO M

8020 A(I,M + 1) = 0: NEXT :A(K,M + 1) = 1: GOSUB 6000:X(K,0) = A(K,M + 1): NEXT : RETURN

8999 REM READ DATA FROM DISK

9000 TEXT : HOME : VTAB 4: PRINT "NONLINEAR REGRESSION ANALYSIS"

9010 PRINT : INPUT "ENTER DATA FILE NAME (PRESS RETURN TO CATALOG DRIVE ONE DISK) ";FI$

9020 IF LEN (FI$) = 0 THEN PRINT CHR$ (4);"CATALOG": GOTO 9010

9030 REM READ DATA FILE

9040 PRINT CHR$ (4);"OPEN ";FI$

9050 PRINT CHR$ (4);"READ ";FI$

9060 INPUT RC,MC,T$

9070 FOR J = 0 TO MC: INPUT RD$(J): NEXT J

9080 PRINT CHR$ (4)

```
9090   PRINT
9100 FOR J = 0 TO MC: PRINT J;")"; TAB( 4);RD$(J): NEXT J
9110 N = RC * LN: DIM TX(N),CY(N),WT(N): REM TX, CY, WT –
     X, Y, AND WEIGHT
9120 FOR I = 1 TO LN
9130 PRINT : PRINT "ENTER # FOR X VARIABLE – LINE ";I;" ";:
     GET T$: PRINT T$:XI(I) = VAL (T$)
9140 IF XI(I) > MC OR XI(I) < 0 THEN GOTO 9130
9150 PRINT "ENTER # FOR Y VARIABLE – LINE ";I;" ";: GET T$:
     PRINT T$:YI(I) = VAL (T$)
9160 IF YI(I) > MC OR YI(I) < 0 THEN GOTO 9150
9170 NEXT I
9180 PRINT : FOR I = 1 TO LN: PRINT "FOR LINE ";I: POKE 36,15:
     PRINT  RD$(YI(I))
9190 PRINT : PRINT TAB( 8);"AS A FUNCTION OF ": PRINT
9200 POKE 36,15: PRINT RD$(XI(I)): PRINT : NEXT I
9210 FOR J = 1 TO LN
9220 NL(J) = RC
9230 NEXT J
9240 PRINT : INPUT "OK SO FAR (Y/N) ";T$: IF T$ < > "Y" AND
     T$ < > "y" THEN PRINT CHR$ (4);"CLOSE ";FI$: RUN
9250 PRINT CHR$ (4);"READ ";FI$
9260 FOR I = 1 TO RC
9270 FOR J = 0 TO MC
9280 INPUT RV$(J)
9290 NEXT J
9300 FOR IJ = 1 TO LN
9310 II = (IJ – 1) * RC + I
9320 TX(II) = VAL (RV$(XI(IJ)))
9330 CY(II) = VAL (RV$(YI(IJ)))
9340 NEXT IJ
9350 NEXT I
9360 PRINT CHR$ (4);"CLOSE ";FI$
9370   RETURN
9999 REM FINAL SS AND R SQUARED
10000 SS = 0:Y1 = 0:Y2 = 0:BS = 0
10010 FOR J = 1 TO LN:BS = BS + NL(J – 1):SL = 0:X1 = 0:X2 = 0
10020 FOR I = 1 TO NL(J):T = TX(BS + I):C = CY(BS + I)
10030 GOSUB 1000
10040 IF C < > 0 THEN SL = SL + (C – CP) ∧ 2 / C ∧ IW
10045 X1 = X1 + C:X2 = X2 + C * C
10050 NEXT I:T = X2 – X1 * X1 / NL(J): PRINT "WSS FOR LINE
      (";J;") IS ";SL;" R SQUARED IS ";(T – SL) / T:SS = SS +
      SL:Y1 = Y1 + X1:Y2 = Y2 + X2
10060 NEXT J:BS = BS + NL(LN):T = Y2 – Y1 * Y1 / BS: PRINT :
      PRINT "TOTAL WSS IS ";SS;" TOTAL R∧2 IS ";(T – SS) / T
10070 IF P$ < > "Y" AND P$ < > "y" THEN PRINT : PRINT
      "PRESS RETURN TO CONTINUE ";: INPUT T$
```

```
10080   RETURN
10999 REM AUC CALCULATION
11000 BS = 0: PRINT
11010 FOR J = 1 TO LN:BS = BS + NL(J - 1):AUC = 0
11020 X1 = TX(BS + 1):Y1 = CY(BS + 1):ST = 2
11030 IF X1 = 0 THEN GOTO 11100
11040 T = 0: GOSUB 1000
11050 ST = 1:X1 = 0:Y1 = CP
11100 FOR I = ST TO NL(J)
11110 X2 = TX(BS + I):Y2 = CY(BS + I)
11120 AUC = AUC + (X2 - X1) * (Y1 + Y2) / 2:X1 = X2:Y1 = Y2:
        NEXT
11130 PRINT "THE AUC FOR LINE (";J;") FROM 0 -> ";TX(BS +
        NL(J));" IS ";AUC
11140 NEXT J: RETURN
11199 REM OUTPUT FOR GRAPHING PROGRAM
11200 PRINT : PRINT "DOES THE DATA DISK HAVE ENOUGH
        SPACE FOR OUTPUT FILES ";: GET T$: PRINT T$
11210 IF T$ < > "y" AND T$ < > "Y" THEN RETURN
11220 PRINT :BS = 0
11230 FOR I = 1 TO LN
11240 FI$ = MID$ (FI$,1, LEN (FI$) - 4) + "(" + STR$ (I) +
        STR$ (AL) + STR$ (IW) + ")" + ".CAL"
11250 PRINT CHR$ (4);"OPEN ";FI$
11260 PRINT CHR$ (4);"WRITE ";FI$
11265 : PRINT "101": PRINT "1": PRINT FI$
11267 PRINT RD$(XI(I)): PRINT RD$(YI(I))
11270 BS = BS + NL(I):X = TX(BS) / 100
11280 FOR J = 0 TO 100
11290 T = J * X: ON I GOSUB 1000,1100,1200,1300,1400
11300 PRINT T: PRINT CP
11310 NEXT J
11320 PRINT CHR$ (4);"CLOSE ";FI$
11330 NEXT I
11340   RETURN
11399 REM MODEL DEFINITION
11400 TEXT : HOME
11410 HTAB 5: PRINT "ONE COMPARTMENT MODELS": PRINT
11420 PRINT "1) RAPID I.V. INJECTION"
11430 PRINT "2) I.V. INFUSION"
11440 PRINT "3) ORAL DOSAGE"
11450 PRINT : HTAB 5: PRINT "TWO COMPARTMENT MODEL":
        PRINT
11460 PRINT "4) RAPID I.V. INJECTION"
11490 PRINT : PRINT "5) YOUR MODEL DEFINED AT 1110-1150":
        PRINT
11500 HTAB 10: INPUT "ENTER CHOICE ";T$
11510 MD = VAL (T$): IF MD < 1 OR MD > 5 THEN 11400
```

```
11520 DIM PL$(9),CN$(9): FOR T = 1 TO 9:PL$(T) = "P(" + STR$
       (T) + ")": NEXT : FOR T = 1 TO 9:CN$(T) = "CN(" + STR$
       (T) + ")": NEXT : IF MD = 5 THEN GOTO 54
11530 LN = 1: DIM NL(LN)
11540 ON MD GOTO 11610,11620,11630,11640
11610 M = 2:NC = 1:PL$(1) = "KEL":PL$(2) = "V":CN$(1) =
       "DOSE":MD$ = "ONE COMPARTMENT-I.V. BOLUS":
       GOTO 11700
11620 M = 2:NC = 2:PL$(1) = "KEL":PL$(2) = "V":CN$(1) =
       "T-INF":CN$(2) = "K0":MD$ = "ONE COMPARTMENT-
       I.V. INFUSION": GOTO 11700
11630 M = 3:NC = 1:PL$(1) = "KEL":PL$(2) = "KA":PL$(3) =
       "V/F":CN$(1) = "DOSE":MD$ = "ONE COMPARTMENT-
       ORAL": GOTO 11700
11640 M = 4:NC = 0:PL$(1) = "A":PL$(2) = "ALPHA":PL$(3) =
       "B":PL$(4) = "BETA":MD$ = "TWO COMPARTMENT-I.V.
       BOLUS": GOTO 11700
11700 GOTO 56
```

GRAPH.IT Program Listing

```
1  REM GRAPH.IT
2  REM BY DAVID WA BOURNE 15 MAY 1985
3  PRINT CHR$ (4);"BLOAD ASCII(36000)":REM ENTERED FROM
       SHAPE TABLE DATA LISTING
4  HIMEM: 35999: LOMEM: 24576
5  POKE 232,160: POKE 233,140
9  GOTO 1000
20 REM S/R TO CHECK X AND Y
21 IF X > 276 THEN X = 276: REM 276=279-3
22 IF X < X0 THEN X = X0
23 IF Y > Y0 THEN Y = Y0
24 IF Y < 3 THEN Y = 3
25   RETURN
30 REM S/R TO SCALE X(I),Y(I) ANSWER IN X,Y
31 X = X(I):Y = Y(I)
32 IF FL% = 0 THEN 35
33 IF Y < S2 THEN Y = S2
34 Y = LOG (Y) / S1
35 X = X0 + X * S3:Y = Y0 + (Y - YL) * S4
36 GOSUB 20
37 PRINT X,Y: RETURN
39 REM S/R TO GRAPH DATA
40 S1 = LOG (10):S2 = EXP (YL * S1):S3 = (X9 - X0) /
       (XH - XL):S4 = (Y9 - Y0) / (YH - YL)
42 IF DF = 1 THEN GOTO 50
44 I = 1: GOSUB 30: HPLOT X,Y
```

```
46 FOR I = 2 TO ND: GOSUB 30: HPLOT TO X,Y: NEXT
48   RETURN
50 FOR I = 1 TO ND: GOSUB 30: HPLOT X + 3,Y + 3: HPLOT TO
     X - 3,Y - 3: HPLOT X + 3,Y - 3: HPLOT TO X - 3,Y + 3:
     NEXT
52   RETURN
100 REM S/R TO PRINT CENTRED TITLE
101 REM T$ = TITLE STRING
102 HTAB (40 - LEN (T$)) / 2: PRINT T$
103   RETURN
110 REM S/R TO INITIALIZE HI-RES PLOTTING
111 HCOLOR= 3: ROT= 0: SCALE= 1
112 HGR : GOSUB 150
113   RETURN
120 REM S/R TO PRINT HORIZONTAL STRING T$ AT X,Y
121 L = LEN (T$): IF L = 0 THEN RETURN : REM NULL STRING
122 FOR I1 = 0 TO L - 1
123 IF X + I1 * 7 > 279 THEN RETURN
124 IF MID$ (T$,I1 + 1,1) = " " THEN GOTO 126
125 XDRAW ASC ( MID$ (T$,I1 + 1,1)) - 31 AT X + I1 * 7,Y
126 NEXT I1
127   RETURN
130 REM S/R TO PRINT VERTICAL STRING
131 ROT= 48:L = LEN (T$): IF L = 0 THEN RETURN
132 FOR I1 = 0 TO L - 1
133 IF Y - I1 * 7 < 0 THEN GOTO 136
134 IF MID$ (T$,I1 + 1,1) = " " THEN GOTO 136
135 DRAW ASC ( MID$ (T$,I1 + 1,1)) - 31 AT X,Y - I1 * 7
136 NEXT I1
137 ROT= 0: RETURN
140 REM S/R TO PUT FOUR LINES ON HI-RES
141 POKE - 16301,0: RETURN
150 REM S/R FULL HI-RES WITHOUT CLEAR
151 POKE - 16304,0: POKE - 16302,0
152   RETURN
160 REM S/R TO CLEAR SCREEN EXCEPT T LINE AT TOP
161 POKE 34,T: HOME : POKE 34,0: RETURN
200 REM S/R TO CREATE DELAY
201 REM T=DELAY STEP
202 FOR I1 = 1 TO T: NEXT I1
203   RETURN
210 REM S/R TO DRAW AXIS
211 X0 = 25:Y0 = 166:X9 = 265:Y9 = 11
212 HPLOT X0,Y0 TO X0,Y9
213 HPLOT X0,Y0 TO X9,Y0
214   RETURN
220 REM S/R TO DRAW HORIZONTAL TICS
221 XT = 6
```

222 FOR I = 0 TO XT
223 HPLOT X0 + (X9 – X0) * I / XT,Y0 + 1 TO X0 + (X9 – X0) * I / XT,Y0 + 3
224 T$ = STR$ (INT ((XL + (XH – XL) * I / XT) * 10 + 0.5) / 10):X = X0 + (X9 – X0) * I / XT + 1.5 – LEN (T$) * 3.5:Y = Y0 + 12: GOSUB 120
225 NEXT I
226 T$ = RD$(XI):X = X0 + (X9 – X0 – 7 * LEN (T$)) / 2:Y = 190: GOSUB 120
227   RETURN
230 REM S/R TO DRAW VERTICAL TICS
231 YT = 5: IF FL% > 0 THEN YT = FL%
232 FOR I = 0 TO YT
233 HPLOT X0 – 1,Y0 + (Y9 – Y0) * I / YT TO X0 – 3,Y0 + (Y9 – Y0) * I / YT
234 T$ = STR$ (INT ((YL + (YH – YL) * I / YT) * 10 + 0.5) / 10):X = X0 – 7:Y = Y0 + (Y9 – Y0) * I / YT – 1.5 + LEN (T$) * 3.5: GOSUB 130
235 NEXT I
236 T$ = RD$(YI): IF FL% < > 0 THEN T$ = "LOG (" + T$ + ")"
237 X = 8:Y = Y0 – (Y0 – Y9 – 7 * LEN (T$)) / 2: GOSUB 130
238   RETURN
240 REM S/R TO SET-UP PLOT
241 GOSUB 210
242 GOSUB 220
243 GOSUB 230
244   RETURN
300 REM S/R TO READ DATA FROM DISK
310 PRINT : PRINT "ENTER DATA FILE NAME (WITH EXTENSION)": PRINT : INPUT FI$: IF FI$ = "" THEN PRINT CHR$ (4);"CATALOG": GOTO 310
320 DF = 1: IF MID$ (FI$, LEN (FI$) – 2,3) = "CAL" THEN DF = 2
330 PRINT CHR$ (4);"OPEN ";FI$: PRINT CHR$ (4);"READ ";FI$
340 INPUT ND,MC,T$
350 FOR J = 0 TO MC: INPUT RD$(J): NEXT J
360 PRINT CHR$ (4)
370 PRINT : FOR J = 0 TO MC: PRINT J;")"; TAB(4);RD$(J): NEXT J
380 PRINT : PRINT "ENTER # FOR X VARIABLE ";: GET T$: PRINT T$:XI = VAL (T$): IF XI > MC OR XI < 0 THEN 380
390 PRINT "ENTER # FOR Y VARIABLE ";: GET T$: PRINT T$:YI = VAL (T$): IF YI > MC OR YI < 0 THEN 390
400 PRINT : PRINT "THUS PLOT IS ";RD$(YI): PRINT : PRINT "AS A FUNCTION OF ";RD$(XI)
410 PRINT : INPUT "OK (Y/N) ";T$: PRINT T$: IF T$ < > "Y" AND T$ < > "y" THEN PRINT CHR$ (4);"CLOSE ";FI$: RUN
420 PRINT CHR$ (4);"READ ";FI$

```
430 FOR I = 1 TO ND: FOR J = 0 TO MC
440 INPUT RV$(J): NEXT J
450 X(I) = VAL (RV$(XI)):Y(I) = VAL (RV$(YI)): NEXT I
460 PRINT CHR$ (4);"CLOSE ";FI$
470   RETURN
500 REM BRANCH TO DRAW NEW LINE
510 ONERR GOTO 500
520 GOSUB 300
530 ONERR GOTO 2000
540 PRINT : PRINT :T$ = "STAND BY FOR PLOT": GOSUB 100
550 T = 250: GOSUB 200
560 GOSUB 150
570 GOTO 4250
1000 REM START OF PROGRAM
1010 REM INITIALIZE PARAMETER ARRAYS
1020 DIM X(101),Y(101)
1030 DF = 0: REM NO DATA YET
2000 REM GREETING FRAME
2005   TEXT
2010 FOR I = 7 TO 1 STEP - 1
2020   HOME
2030 VTAB I: INVERSE :T$ = "** GRAPH.IT, A PLOTTING
        PROGRAM **": GOSUB 100: NORMAL
2040 VTAB I * 2:T$ = "DEPARTMENT OF PHARMACY": GOSUB
        100
2050 VTAB I * 3:T$ = "UNIVERSITY OF QUEENSLAND": GOSUB
        100
2060 T = 200: GOSUB 200
2070 NEXT I
2080 POKE - 16368,0
3000 REM INSTRUCTIONS
3010 PRINT : PRINT
4000 REM DISPLAY OPTIONS AND GET INPUT
4010 HOME : PRINT
4020 INVERSE :T$ = "** GRAPH.IT **": GOSUB 100: NORMAL
4030 PRINT : PRINT : PRINT :T$ = "ENTER MAXIMUM VALUE
        OF X (TIME)": GOSUB 100
4040 PRINT :T$ = "(MULTIPLES OF 6 ARE BEST)": GOSUB 100
4050 PRINT : HTAB 19: INPUT T$:XH = VAL (T$)
4060 IF XH > 0 GOTO 4080
4070 PRINT :T$ = "MUST BE GREATER THAN ZERO": GOSUB
        100: GOTO 4030
4080 XL = 0
4100 PRINT : PRINT : PRINT :T$ = "FOR SEMI-LOG PLOT, ENTER
        # OF CYCLES": GOSUB 100
4110 T$ = "ENTER 0 FOR LINEAR PLOT": GOSUB 100
4120 HTAB 19: INPUT T$:FL% = VAL (T$)
4130 IF FL% < 6 AND FL% > = 0 THEN GOTO 4150
```

```
4140 PRINT :T$ = "MUST BE BETWEEN 0 AND 5 INCLUSIVE":
     GOSUB 100: GOTO 4100
4150 IF FL% > 0 THEN GOTO 4180
4160 REM  LINEAR  TRACK
4161 PRINT : PRINT : PRINT :T$ = "ENTER MAXIMUM VALUE
     OF Y (CONC.)": GOSUB 100
4162 PRINT :T$ = "(MULTIPLES OF 5 ARE BEST)": GOSUB 100
4163 PRINT : HTAB 19: INPUT T$:YH = VAL (T$)
4164 IF YH > 0 GOTO 4166
4165 PRINT :T$ = "MUST BE GREATER THAN ZERO": GOSUB
     100: GOTO 4160
4166 YL = 0
4179 GOTO  4210
4180 REM  SEMI-LOG  TRACK
4181 PRINT : PRINT : PRINT :T$ = "ENTER MAXIMUM VALUE
     OF Y (CONC.)": GOSUB 100
4182 PRINT :T$ = "(MUST BE EVEN POWER OF 10)": GOSUB 100
4183 PRINT : HTAB 18: INPUT T$: IF VAL (T$) < = 0 THEN PRINT
     :T$ = "MUST BE POSITIVE AND NOT ZERO": GOSUB 100:
     GOTO  4180
4184 YH = LOG ( VAL (T$)) / LOG (10): IF YH = INT (YH) GOTO
     4186
4185 PRINT :T$ = "MUST BE .1, 1, 10, OR 100 etc": GOSUB 100:
     GOTO  4180
4186 YL = YH – FL%
4210 IF DF < > 0 THEN 4220
4212 ONERR  GOTO  4210
4214 GOSUB  300
4216 ONERR  GOTO  2000
4220 PRINT : PRINT :T$ = "STAND BY FOR PLOT": GOSUB 100
4230 T = 250: GOSUB 200
4240 GOSUB 110: GOSUB 240
4250 GOSUB 40
4260 PRINT CHR$ (7): GET T$: PRINT CHR$ (7)
4270 T = 20: GOSUB 160
4280 GOSUB  140
4290 VTAB 21:T$ = "ENTER CHOICE": INVERSE : GOSUB 100:
     NORMAL
4300 VTAB 22:T$ = "1) NEW DATA 2) NEW AXES 3) PRINT":
     GOSUB  100
4305 T$ = "4) EXIT": GOSUB 100
4310 HTAB 19: INPUT T$:T = VAL (T$)
4320 IF T > 4 OR T < 1 THEN GOTO 4300
4321 T = 0: GOSUB 160
4330 T = VAL (T$): TEXT
4340 IF T = 1 THEN GOTO 500
4350 IF T = 2 THEN GOTO 4000
4355 IF T = 3 THEN GOTO 4500
```

4360 T$ = "RETURNING TO MENU": FLASH : GOSUB 100:
     NORMAL
4370 PRINT CHR$ (4);"RUN HELLO,D1"
4380 END
4500 REM PRINTER PLOT SECTION – FOR EPSON FX-80+ AND
     PRACTICAL PERIPHERALS MICROBUFFER INTERFACE
     CARD
4510 PRINT "LAST FILE NAME WAS – ";FI$
4520 INPUT "ENTER TITLE FOR PLOT ";TI$
4530 PRINT CHR$ (4);"PR#1
4540 PRINT TAB(40 – LEN (TI$) / 2);TI$
4550 PRINT CHR$ (9);"GE"
4570 PRINT : PRINT : PRINT CHR$ (4);"PR#0"
4580 PRINT : PRINT : PRINT : PRINT : PRINT
4590 GOTO 4290

Shape Table Data

```
8CA0 - 5B 00  B8 00  BE 00  C5 00  CE 00  E0 00  F0 00  FC 00
8CB0 - 0C 01  14 01  1C 01  26 01  34 01  3D 01  41 01  47 01
8CC0 - 4A 01  50 01  5B 01  62 01  71 01  7D 01  8A 01  96 01
8CD0 - A4 01  AC 01  BB 01  C8 01  CF 01  D5 01  DE 01  E8 01
8CE0 - F0 01  FA 01  07 02  14 02  21 02  2B 02  36 02  42 02
8CF0 - 4B 02  57 02  64 02  6C 02  74 02  81 02  89 02  97 02
8D00 - A3 02  AE 02  B7 02  C3 02  CF 02  DC 02  E4 02  EF 02
8D10 - FC 02  08 03  13 03  1C 03  28 03  31 03  3B 03  43 03
8D20 - 4B 03  4F 03  59 03  63 03  6D 03  76 03  81 03  8B 03
8D30 - 94 03  A1 03  AA 03  B2 03  BD 03  C8 03  CF 03  D8 03
8D40 - DE 03  E7 03  F1 03  FB 03  03 04  0D 04  18 04  20 04
8D50 - 2B 04  36 04  40 04  4C 04  3E 24  2D 36  04 00  09 0C
8D60 - 18 24  24 04  00 09  18 08  18 20  6C 36  04 00  08 18
8D70 - 2D 2D  0C 18  3F 3F  0C 58  B6 16  6E 24  20 20  04 00
8D80 - 28 2D  0D 18  1C 3F  0F 18  0C 2D  E5 B3  16 16  04 00
8D90 - 60 0C  0C 0C  DF 27  B5 92  09 35  27 00  20 0C  0D 18
8DA0 - E4 17  B6 09  15 15  0C 18  9F 3A  04 00  09 08  18 08
8DB0 - 18 24  04 00  09 1C  1C 24  0C 0C  04 00  09 0D  18 0D
8DC0 - 18 24  1C 1C  04 00  60 0C  0C 0C  DC 36  16 36  0D E0
8DD0 - DC E0  04 00  08 18  28 2D  25 D8  B6 26  00 29  20 04
8DE0 - 00 08  18 28  2D 25  00 09  04 00  60 0C  0C 0C  04 00
8DF0 - 09 0D  18 24  24 1C  17 36  36 04  00 29  E5 24  24 BC
8E00 - 04 00  2D 2D  0C 18  08 18  E4 3F  17 96  2A 28  28 04
8E10 - 00 A8  2D 0D  18 E4  67 0D  18 3C  3F 27  00 08  18 64
8E20 - 0C 0C  36 36  36 0D  18 F8  27 00  A8 2D  0D 18  24 1C
8E30 - 3F 27  2C 2D  25 00  20 24  0C 0C  2D 96  32 1E  3F 0C
8E40 - 18 28  25 00  21 64  0C 0C  3C 3F  27 00  20 0C  2D 0D
8E50 - 18 E4  3F 17  B6 49  31 1E  3F 04  00 2D  0D 18  0D 18
8E60 - 24 E4  3F 17  76 2D  04 00  09 08  18 0C  18 04  00 29
```

```
8E70 -  20 0C 18 04 00 49 1C 1C 1C 0C 0C 0C 04 00 08 18
8E80 -  2D 2D 0C 18 3F 3F 04 00 29 28 28 E0 1C 1C 04 00
8E90 -  09 0C 18 64 0C 1C 3F 17 04 00 E1 24 24 0C 2D 15
8EA0 -  36 3F B4 16 2D 04 00 24 24 0C 0C 15 15 36 36 0F
8EB0 -  18 38 27 00 24 24 24 2D AD F6 3F 96 2D 0D 18 24
8EC0 -  00 20 24 64 2D 15 96 F2 3F 04 00 24 24 24 2D AD
8ED0 -  36 36 1E 3F 04 00 24 24 24 2D 2D 96 3B B7 2A 2D
8EE0 -  04 00 24 24 24 2D 2D 96 3B 27 00 20 24 64 2D B5
8EF0 -  12 FF 12 2D 25 04 00 24 24 24 4D 31 36 36 3E 08
8F00 -  18 38 27 00 29 E5 24 24 3C 0D 04 00 A8 2D 0D 18
8F10 -  24 24 24 00 24 24 24 95 2A 28 28 B0 D2 73 0E 04
8F20 -  00 2D 2D DC 1B 24 24 24 00 24 24 24 15 15 2E 08
8F30 -  18 0C 36 36 36 04 00 24 24 24 95 0E 0E 56 24 24
8F40 -  24 04 00 20 24 64 2D 15 36 36 1E 3F 04 00 24 24
8F50 -  24 2D AD F6 3F 04 00 20 24 64 2D 15 36 FE 0E 0E
8F60 -  1F 27 00 24 24 24 2D AD F6 3F 0E 0E 0E 04 00 A8
8F70 -  2D 0D 18 E4 3F 0F 18 64 2D 15 04 00 09 24 24 24
8F80 -  3F 4D 25 00 20 24 24 4D 31 36 36 1E 3F 04 00 08
8F90 -  18 24 24 4D 31 36 F6 1E 0F 18 04 00 24 24 24 4D
8FA0 -  31 36 36 3E 38 B8 04 00 64 0C 0C 0C FC 1B 76 56
8FB0 -  71 26 00 09 24 64 0C FC 1B 76 04 00 64 0C 0C 0C
8FC0 -  3C 3F B7 92 0A 2D 25 00 49 3F 27 24 24 2C 2D 04
8FD0 -  00 08 18 08 18 70 0E 0E 0E 04 00 29 2D 24 24 24
8FE0 -  3F 27 00 08 18 60 0C 0E 0E 04 00 2D 2D 04 00 08
8FF0 -  18 08 18 08 58 A9 15 04 00 60 2D 25 1C 3F 96 2A
9000 -  2D 24 00 24 24 24 95 2A AD F6 3F 04 00 49 3F 0F
9010 -  18 24 0C 2D 04 00 20 0C 2D 25 24 96 32 3E 3F 04
9020 -  00 20 64 2D 15 3E 3F 16 2D 25 00 21 24 24 0C AD
9030 -  D6 FF 04 00 20 0C 2D 15 36 36 1E 3F 0C 18 28 25
9040 -  00 24 24 24 95 2A AD 36 04 00 29 E5 24 3C 0C 58
9050 -  04 00 52 15 0D 18 24 24 3C 0C 58 04 00 24 24 24
9060 -  95 12 0C 0C 96 73 04 00 29 E5 24 24 3C 04 00 24
9070 -  64 15 36 6E 24 E4 04 00 24 64 AD 36 26 00 20 64
9080 -  2D 15 36 1E 3F 04 00 24 2C 2D 15 F6 3F 17 36 04
9090 -  00 20 0C 2D 36 3E 77 31 2E 20 00 24 24 15 0D 18
90A0 -  15 04 00 2D 2D E0 3F 0F 18 0C 2D 25 00 49 09 18
90B0 -  17 3F 20 24 BC 0D 25 00 20 24 4D 36 76 1F 27 00
90C0 -  08 18 24 4D 31 F6 1E 0F 18 04 00 20 24 4D 31 36
90D0 -  1E 0F 18 BC 22 00 0C 0C 0C 0C DF 73 56 71 04 00
90E0 -  20 6C 09 36 36 F6 3F 0C 18 28 25 00 0C 0C 0C 0C
90F0 -  3F 3F 96 0A 2D 25 00
```

Index

Printed in the United Kingdom
by Lightning Source UK Ltd.
115489UKS00006B/264